The bad news: Hypertension affects an estimated fifty million Americans and countless millions worldwide. It is the most significant predisposing factor for heart attack, stroke, and peripheral artery disease—and, left untreated, gradually destroys the heart, blood vessels, and kidneys. To make matters worse, doctors often overmedicate patients with expensive and sometimes dangerous drugs.

The good news: Ninety-five percent of all hypertension is controllable. Featuring a concise and effective program, this book will help you to take charge of your health, prevent the factors that lead to hypertension, and most likely decrease your dependence on drugs that may have dangerous side effects. . . even if your high blood pressure requires immediate attention. Guidance on diet, exercise, mineral supplements, water intake, stress management, and fabulous recipes too—here is everything you need to begin. . .

REVERSING HYPERTENSION

"Might be just what the doctor ordered . . . recommended."

—Library Journal

Also by Julian Whitaker, M.D., and Warner Books

Reversing Heart Disease
Reversing Diabetes

REVERSING
HYPERTENSION

A VITAL NEW PROGRAM TO PREVENT, TREAT, AND REDUCE HIGH BLOOD PRESSURE

JULIAN WHITAKER, M.D.

**WELLNESS
CENTRAL**

NEW YORK   BOSTON

Copyright © 2000 by Julian Whitaker, M.D.

Wellness Central
Hachette Book Group
237 Park Avenue
New York, NY 10017

Visit our Web site at www.HachetteBookGroup.com.

Printed in the United States of America

Originally published in hardcover by Hachette Book Group.
First Trade Edition: February 2001
10   9   8

Wellness Central is an imprint of Grand Central Publishing.
The Wellness Central name and logo are trademarks of Hachette Book Group, Inc.

The Library of Congress has cataloged the hardcover edition as follows:
Whitaker, Julian M.
    Reversing hypertension : a vital new program to prevent, treat, and reduce high blood pressure / Julian Whitaker.
        p.   cm.
    Includes bibliographical references and index.
    ISBN 0-446-52286-4
    1. Hypertension—Popular works.   2. Hypertension—Diet therapy.
3. Dietary supplements.   I. Title.
    RC685.H8W47   2000
    616.1'32—dc21
                                                     99-39815
                                                        CIP

ISBN 978-0-446-67663-2 (pbk.)

Cover design by Flag

For all the readers of this book,
with my sincerest wishes for a long and healthy life.

Contents

Acknowledgments

I would like to acknowledge several people for their significant contributions to this book, particularly my research director, Peggy Dace, and Mia Simms, who did much of the initial research. I would also like to thank Kelley Griffin for her proofreading and editing, Marida Hines for her illustrations, and Diana Baroni, my editor at Warner Books. Finally, for her love, support, and inspiration, I owe a debt of gratitude to my wife, Connie.

Introduction

Some twenty-five years ago, I decided to take "the road less traveled" in medicine. I was a young physician, ardent about my profession but disillusioned by what lay down the well-trodden path of conventional medicine. All I could see in my future were prescription pads and surgical procedures, and I knew there had to be a better way. I embraced the new principles of healing discussed in this book—which I learned only after graduating from medical school—with such passion that I knew I had to share them with my patients. I also knew that it was impossible to do this in a ten-minute office visit. I wanted to get involved with my patients, to help them understand the power of natural therapies, and how to utilize these therapies to heal themselves.

My dream was to have a clinic where patients could come together as a group for one or two weeks and, through a program of education and hands-on lifestyle changes, get well. Having worked with nutrition pioneer Nathan Pritikin, I knew such a program would work. And I was sure that tangible improvements in their condition, along with the support of fellow patients, would be powerful motivation for patients to stick with the program—and continue to get better—once they returned home. So in 1979 I opened the doors to the Whitaker Wellness Institute. Eight patients enrolled in my fledgling clinic to undergo two weeks of lifestyle restructuring, focusing on diet, exercise, stress management, and vitamin and mineral supplementation. Twenty-plus years later we're still going strong.

Over that time we have treated thousands of patients with serious, life-threatening conditions such as hypertension, heart disease, and diabetes. In many cases they have come to us as a last resort, after conventional medicine had given up on them. Yet when patients live the healthy lifestyle I prescribe—even for so little a time as one week—miraculous things begin to happen. Blood pressure plummets. Exercise endurance improves. Weight goes down. Medications are discontinued. Aches and pains ease. All in one short week! The really exciting stuff, however, happens after patients go home. Armed with hope, information, and newfound resolve, they find that they are able to stick with this program, and they continue to improve.

It is out of these weeklong clinics that my program for reversing hypertension, the one presented in this book, has evolved. For more than twenty-five years I've closely monitored thousands of patients with hypertension. I've followed them for months and even years after they've gone through the program. This has given me a feel for what works over the long term, as well as what lifestyle changes patients are willing to make. I've also pored over the medical literature, examining volumes of research studies, and added new elements to the program as they have proven effective.

My patients have been my teachers, and it is the lessons learned from them and with them that are presented in this book. Throughout these pages you will read about people who have embraced this program and reversed their hypertension. It is my sincerest desire that you achieve similar results, so that you can enjoy optimal health—and live life to its fullest.

Julian M. Whitaker, M.D.

REVERSING HYPERTENSION

PART I

⌄

HYPERTENSION AND ITS RELATED RISKS

Nicole came to the Whitaker Wellness Institute "to get my life back." She had just turned 50 and was overweight with severe fluid retention. She was depressed, unable to sleep, and she ached all over. She had no energy and was so lethargic that she spent most of her days just sitting in a chair. She had been diagnosed with hypertension some years earlier, but since the medication prescribed disagreed with her, she had stopped taking it.

When Nicole's blood pressure was taken during her initial examination, it was a sky-high 210/110 mm Hg. Her heart was enlarged and unable to pump efficiently, a hallmark of untreated hypertension. Nicole was started on a comprehensive nutritional supplement program, along with a course of medication to reduce her fluid retention and bring her dangerously high blood pressure down immediately. She was encouraged to begin a walking program, starting with only 5 minutes a day—which was all she could handle initially—and building up as she regained strength and energy. She was also advised to make dramatic changes in her diet. Nicole was so desperately ill that she agreed to try anything.

Over the next few months, Nicole returned to my office regularly. Within two months she had lost 32 pounds and her blood pressure was down to 132/94. After four months she was down another 12 pounds, her blood pressure had fallen to 128/84, and we began to slowly wean her off medication. Nicole wrote this note: "I no longer have a constant ache in my back. I sleep like a log, usually no less than six hours and up to eight hours. I am up to 15 minutes on the treadmill. Stairs no longer present a problem for me. Actually, I haven't even been winded after climbing three flights of stairs. I have come a long way from sitting in a chair for the better part of five months. Thank you for your expertise, intellect, and caring."

Hypertension, or high blood pressure, is a silent killer. It places tremendous stress on the arteries and overworks the heart with each beat. Hypertension may progress for years without symptoms, slowly chipping away at the blood vessels, heart, and kidneys. And it eventually takes its toll—high blood pressure is the major underlying cause of heart attacks and strokes. Conventional treatment is sometimes worse than the disease, as patients with hypertension are often overmedicated with prescription drugs that have unpleasant side effects. Even if these drugs do lower blood pressure, they may significantly decrease quality of life and increase the risk of other health problems, while doing little to prevent cardiovascular complications.

Though many doctors still define hypertension as "causeless" or of "unknown origin," don't buy it. Extensive medical research, which I will tell you about in this book, makes it perfectly clear that unhealthy living is the primary cause of hypertension. And while it's true that age, race, and genetic and environmental factors can put you at increased risk, your daily habits do far more to determine whether or not you will develop this condition. This is great news, for it means that preventing and reversing hypertension are within your control.

I've spent more than twenty-five years treating patients with hypertension and have found that the human body responds rapidly when nurtured and given a chance to heal itself. Like Nicole, hundreds of patients treated at the Whitaker Wellness Institute have lowered their blood pressure using safe, effective, natural therapies. This book offers you the same sensible program I offer patients at my clinic. *Reversing Hypertension* is your complete guide to regaining and maintaining normal blood pressure for life. In Part I I'll explain exactly how blood pressure is maintained, what drives it up, and how hypertension affects your overall health. We will discuss the drugs commonly prescribed to lower blood pressure, how they work, and how some of these drugs can increase your risk of premature death. Most important, in the detailed program laid out in Part II, you'll learn how to prevent and reverse hypertension by addressing its root causes.

I strongly encourage you to work with your physician as you implement the elements of this program for reversing hypertension. If your doctor is new to natural approaches to medicine, you may wish to share the information in this book with him or her. However, if your physician does not support your desire to utilize these safe nutritional and lifestyle approaches, I suggest you find one who will. (See Appendix E for resources to help you find a doctor knowledgeable in the therapies discussed in this book.)

It is important for you to know that 90 to 95 percent of all hypertension cases can be treated. And an estimated 80 percent of patients with high blood pressure have what is classified as mild to moderate hypertension, which can often be managed through diet, nutritional supplementation, exercise, and stress management. By taking full responsibility for your health and making a few changes in the things you do every day, you can turn you health—and your life—around. Let's get started!

▼ | IF YOUR BLOOD PRESSURE IS DANGEROUSLY HIGH

If your blood pressure is severely high (systolic over 180 mm Hg or diastolic over 110 mm Hg), turn immediately to the Quick Start Diet in Chapter 11. Time is of the essence! Under your physician's supervision, follow the instructions for bringing down blood pressure fast, and watch your blood pressure safely drop to healthy levels. Then go back and read this book from beginning to end to get a good grasp of the causes of and solutions for hypertension. If you've been diagnosed with less severe hypertension, or if you are interested in preventing hypertension, I suggest you take the time to read through the entire book, making the recommended changes as they apply to you.

CHAPTER 1

Hypertension: Action Alert

Hypertension affects an estimated 50 million Americans—more than one in three American adults. It is the lit fuse of a bomb waiting to go off. Hypertension triples your risk of dying from a heart attack and increases your risk of stroke sevenfold over someone with normal blood pressure. Yet hypertension is largely symptom-free—until it's too late. Hypertension is classified as a cardiovascular disease (CVD), a disorder afflicting the heart or blood vessels. According to 1999 American Heart Association (AHA) statistics, 58.8 million Americans suffer one or more of the cardiovascular diseases, making CVD an epidemic of unbelievable proportions. CVD mortality rates actually outrank our country's next seven leading causes of death *combined* (including cancer). Every year 959,227 Americans die of CVD. That's 2,600 per day, or 1 every 33 seconds, which accounts for 41.4 percent of the total deaths in the United States. Imagine, nearly half of all Americans will die from cardiovascular disease—and hypertension is a primary contributor to many of these deaths. If you don't take control of and effectively manage your blood pressure, it will take control of you.

▼ | **ESTIMATED NUMBER OF AMERICANS SUFFERING FROM CARDIOVASCULAR DISEASE**

- Cardiovascular disease (all types): 58.8 million
- Hypertension: 50 million
- Coronary heart disease: 12 million
- Stroke: 4.4 million
- Rheumatic heart disease: 1.8 million
- 1 in 5 Americans have some type of CVD
- 1 in 3 men and 1 in 10 women will develop major CVD before age 60
- 31.6 percent of Americans with hypertension don't know they have it

Source: 1999 American Heart Association statistics.

Although hypertension is extremely common, it is painless and usually symptom-free.

Hypertension does occasionally give subtle warning signs. You might, for example, experience troublesome headaches. These are usually located in the back of the head and upper neck and are most acute in the morning, when blood pressure is relatively low. Vision problems, dizziness, fatigue, abnormal sweating, insomnia, shortness of breath, and excessive flushing of the face are other symptoms you might experience. Any one or a combination of these might signal hypertension. Although these symptoms could also stem from other conditions, if you are experiencing any of them I urge you to consult your physician immediately and have your blood pressure monitored.

Many people with hypertension are completely unaware that they have this insidious condition: of the 50 million Americans with hypertension, only 68.4 percent are aware that their blood pressure is high. This is why I recommend that everyone over age 35 have their blood pressure checked regularly. Although hypertension can strike at any age, blood pressure tends to increase steadily with age, so regular checkups become even more important as you get older.

MEASURING BLOOD PRESSURE

Having your blood pressure checked is quick and painless. It is usually done with a stethoscope and a sphygmomanometer (*sphygmo* means "pulse"), which consists of an inflatable arm cuff attached to a column of mercury and a gauge (see Figure 1). Although newer technologies in monitoring—including wrist and finger cuffs with digital readouts—are becoming more and more popular for home and clinic use, the sphygmomanometer remains the standard.

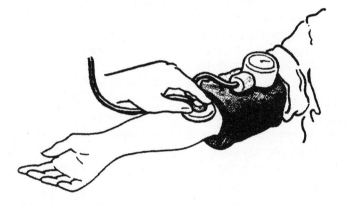

Figure 1. Taking Blood Pressure with a Sphygmomanometer

Here's how a sphygmomanometer works. The cuff, which is wrapped around the upper arm just above the elbow, is inflated with air to compress the brachial artery, the major artery in the arm. The cuff is first inflated to a pressure that shuts off all of the blood flow through the artery. As the cuff is slowly deflated, the person taking the blood pressure reading listens through a stethoscope placed on the brachial artery for the first audible beat—the sound of blood rushing back into the compressed artery—and notes the number on the gauge. (A computer chip in the electronic versions does this for you.) This indicates the *systolic* blood pressure, or pressure generated by the heart immediately after it contracts, or beats, and represents the top number of the blood pressure reading.

As pressure from the cuff continues to be released, the beats become stronger and more distinct, then taper off and disappear. The number at which the last beat is audible indicates the *diastolic* pressure, or the arterial pressure maintained between heartbeats, when the heart is at rest. The combined ratio of systolic over diastolic reveals the relative pressure generated by the heart as it alternately pumps blood through the arteries and rests. The fraction is expressed in millimeters of mercury (mm Hg), which refers to the amount of mercury displaced by the arterial pressure during the reading. So a blood pressure reading of 120/80 mm Hg represents a systolic pressure of 120 and a diastolic pressure of 80.

A blood pressure reading will indicate one of three states: *hypotension* (low blood pressure), *normotension* (normal blood pressure), or *hypertension* (high blood pressure). Normotension is, of course, the ideal. In fact, it's one of the best predictors of a long life. Low blood pressure may not be entirely desirable, but because it is relatively rare, it will not be discussed in this book. If the reading indicates hypertension, your health *is* in danger, and you need to take immediate steps to bring your blood pressure down to healthier levels.

MAKING THE DIAGNOSIS

There is general agreement that optimal blood pressure is 120/80 or less. However, exactly what blood pressure constitutes hypertension is subject to some interpretation. In the past a diagnosis of hypertension was often based exclusively on diastolic blood pressure (the bottom number in the blood pressure reading). If your diastolic pressure was over 90, you had high blood pressure. It was felt that because the heart takes longer to rest than it does to beat, the diastolic measurement was more significant. However, more recent research has made it clear that an elevated diastolic pressure is no more hazardous than a high systolic reading—and the latter appears to be an even more accurate predictor of cardiovascular risk. The current consensus is that elevations in either systolic or diastolic blood pressure readings should be taken seriously. This is particularly true among older people, who may have dangerously high systolic readings while maintaining virtually normal diastolic blood pressure.

According to current American Heart Association guidelines, hypertension is clinically defined as a systolic blood pressure greater than 140 or a diastolic pressure greater than 90. This echoes the recommendations of the Joint National Committee on the Prevention, Detection, Evaluation, and Treatment of High Blood Pressure (JNC), a widely respected National Institutes of Health task force of physicians who are experts in hypertension and whose recommendations are approved by most major organizations. The JNC, which updates its recommendations periodically, published its sixth and latest report of guidelines in November 1997. The committee devised an updated system of diagnosis using both systolic and diastolic blood pressures to assess a patient's health risk. The guidelines also recommend that clinicians specify other known risk factors, including smoking, immoderate drinking, and routine overeating. All of this information is then combined to determine the stage of risk for a specific patient. The higher the stage, the greater the patient's risk of a heart attack or stroke.

▼ | BLOOD PRESSURE CLASSIFICATION

Classification	Systolic (mm Hg)	Diastolic (mm Hg)
Optimal	under 120	under 80
Normal	under 130	under 85
High normal	130–139	85–89
Stage 1 hypertension (Mild)	140–159	90–99
Stage 2 hypertension (Moderate)	160–179	100–109
Stage 3 hypertension (Severe)	180+	110+

Source: JNC VI.

However, more recent research suggests that blood pressure readings for a diagnosis of hypertension might need to be adjusted downward. In June 1998, results of the Hypertension Optimal Treatment (HOT) trial, a five-year study involving almost 19,000 patients from

26 countries, were published in *The Lancet*, one of the world's leading medical journals. Researchers found that patients who were able to lower their systolic blood pressure to an average of 138.5 mm Hg and their diastolic blood pressure to an average of 82.6 had major reductions in heart attack and stroke risk. In early 1999, the World Health Organization and the International Society of Hypertension recommended that the upper limit for high normal blood pressure be lower, 130/85 (down from the JNC's upper limit of 139/89). They based this on findings of the HOT trial and other studies showing that stroke and heart attack risk are dramatically reduced when diastolic blood pressure is less than 85.

You may be thinking, "Why quibble over such small numbers? What's the difference between 85 and 89?" According to an article published in the *Journal of the American Medical Association* in March 1999, a decrease in diastolic blood pressure of only 5 to 6 points lowers your risk for stroke 42 percent.

So when should you be concerned about your blood pressure? Since risk factors decrease as blood pressure goes down, I'd have to agree with the most recent findings. If your blood pressure is above 130/85, you should institute the measures outlined in this book for reversing hypertension and aim to get into the optimal range of 120/80 or lower.

CHECK AND RECHECK YOUR BLOOD PRESSURE

If you have high blood pressure based on a blood pressure reading in your doctor's office, don't panic. Before a true diagnosis is made you should return to the clinic on at least three separate occasions (six return visits for monitoring are even better), so your doctor can evaluate whether your blood pressure is consistently elevated. Your blood pressure changes constantly throughout the day, depending on your environment, activities, diet, emotions, medication, and other factors. Even so simple a thing as talking can dramatically raise your blood pressure. In a 1998 study carried out at the Clinique Cardiologique in Paris, researchers measured the blood pressures of 50 patients with hypertension while they were actively talking, silently reading, or sitting quietly. During the talking period blood pressure significantly increased—by an average of 17 mm Hg systolic and 13 mm Hg diastolic—and it remained elevated, although to a lesser degree, for a time afterward. Silent reading actually lowered blood pressure more than did merely sitting quietly.

Another cause of elevated blood pressure readings—in the absence of true hypertension—is what is known as "white-coat hypertension." For many people, visiting a doctor is stressful, and the sheer anxiety of being examined by a health professional temporarily elevates blood pressure. When this reaction occurs, an inexperienced or hasty medical practitioner may misdiagnose the patient as having hypertension solely on the basis of one or two in-office blood pressure readings. White-coat hypertension is an all-too-common phenomenon that can result in expensive, unnecessary, and potentially hazardous treatment. Despite frequent and supposedly accurate measurements of blood pressure, as many as 12 million patients in the United States may be misclassified as hypertensive.

For this reason, I turn to a test called the twenty-four-hour ambulatory blood pressure monitoring (ABPM) system. This device measures blood pressure every fifteen to thirty minutes and can help determine if a patient has true hypertension. The computerized ABPM monitor is about the size of a paperback book and is attached to a blood pressure cuff. The cuff is worn around the patient's arm, while the monitor is worn on a belt around the waist or over the shoulder like a purse. While the ABPM can take blood pressure readings over a twenty-four-hour period, I have my patients wear it for just twelve to eighteen hours, since I don't want to rob them of a night's sleep. This still gives me the information I need for an accurate evaluation of their blood pressure, allowing me to rule out white-coat hypertension and treat only those patients with true hypertension.

Unfortunately, the overwhelming majority of patients are still being diagnosed with hypertension based solely on a few readings taken in a doctor's office. I feel this is a grave mistake. The authors of a 1993 *Journal of the American Medical Association* study reported that as many as "twenty-one percent of the patients diagnosed as having borderline [high normal] hypertension in the clinic were found to have normal blood pressure readings on ambulatory monitoring." And the sad part about it is that many of these perfectly normal patients are needlessly placed on prescription medications that might actually make them sick.

▼ GUIDELINES FOR HAVING YOUR BLOOD PRESSURE TAKEN

Here are a few things to consider when having your blood pressure taken in your doctor's office to ensure the most accurate readings.

- Don't drink coffee or other caffeine-containing beverages or foods for a couple of hours before your blood pressure is monitored.
- Abstain from smoking for at least thirty minutes prior.
- Don't talk during the reading.
- Request at least two readings, separated by two minutes, one taken in each arm.

If you really want to stay on top of things, I suggest you take your own blood pressure at home. Self-monitoring is easy, economical, and, once you get the hang of it, quite accurate. You could purchase your own sphygmomanometer and stethoscope, which would allow you to take your blood pressure at home anytime. Or contact your local pharmacy or fitness facility and ask if they offer a blood pressure monitoring unit you can use free of charge. (See Appendix D for detailed instructions on measuring your blood pressure with a sphygmomanometer.) Electronic blood pressure monitors are also available. Whatever type of device you choose, take it with you to your next doctor's appointment, so your physician can make sure you are using it properly and it is giving you accurate readings. Remember, although self-monitoring is a viable means of keeping track of your blood pressure, you should do it in conjunction with the professional monitoring and guidance provided by your own physician. Self-monitoring should *not* be used for self-diagnosis.

WHAT DO YOU DO IF YOU HAVE HYPERTENSION?

Once a diagnosis of hypertension is firmly established, what do you do? According to a study entitled "Heartstyles: Profiles in Hypertension," based on data analyzed by Dr. Michael Weber of the State University of New York and his colleagues, you might have one of several reactions. These researchers surveyed 727 patients and came up with four distinct responses to the diagnosis of hypertension.

- The *Actively Attentives* (39 percent of the patients) were the ideal patients. Proactively involved in their health, they educated themselves about their condition and were highly motivated to modify their diets and make other lifestyle changes in an effort to reduce risk factors.
- The *Nonchalant Newcomers* (23 percent) were more difficult. They essentially refused to take their diagnosis seriously. They had limited knowledge about hypertension and made little effort to learn more. They might take medication, but only to pacify their physician.
- The *Honestly Overwhelmed* (22 percent) were the most difficult group. They tended to have lots of problems in their lives and were unable to really focus on the seriousness of their condition. They knew little about hypertension and had few resources.
- The *Mainly Meds* (16 percent) had no motivation to make lifestyle changes, but they were compliant with medications.

If you've gone to the trouble to purchase and read this book, you likely fall into the Actively Attentive group. You're looking for something other than a lifelong dependency on prescription drugs. You understand the implications of hypertension, and you're taking steps to educate yourself about your condition. Furthermore, you probably have the initiative and willpower necessary to make the lifestyle changes that we will discuss in Part II to lower your blood pressure and reduce your risk factors for serious cardiovascular disease. It is for you Actively Attentives that I have written this book.

But before we get into the details of my program for reversing hypertension, let's take a quick lesson in physiology and biochemistry so you will understand exactly what causes hypertension.

CHAPTER 2

Understanding Blood Pressure

With what words will you describe this heart, so as not to fill a book . . . ?

Leonardo da Vinci

Hypertension is generally attributed to persistent tightening of the arterioles, the small blood vessels that branch off the arteries. But this is like saying that flipping a switch turns on the lights, or watering a seed makes it grow—it's only part of the picture. In this chapter we're going to take an in-depth look at blood pressure and the organs and systems involved in its regulation. We'll discuss the heart and blood vessels, which are obviously the primary players in hypertension. We'll also look at other systems that are involved in blood pressure regulation. Your kidneys play a key role, as do your adrenal and pituitary glands and your nervous system. So let's begin our exploration of the inside story of blood pressure. I'll do my best to simplify this very complex subject—and I promise "not to fill a book."

THE PUMP AND PIPES OF THE CARDIOVASCULAR SYSTEM

To describe the cardiovascular system and the basics of blood pressure, I like to use a model that most everyone is familiar with—plumbing. While this analogy may be overly simplistic, your cardiovascular system is essentially a network consisting of a pump and multiple pipes. Your heart is the pump, your blood vessels a complex set of pipes, and your blood the fluid coursing through the system.

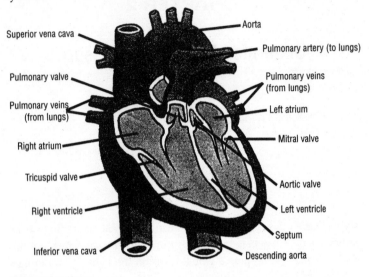

Figure 2. Your Heart

The Pump

What a pump your heart is! About the size of a fist, this muscular organ contracts and relaxes from 50 to 200 times per minute without rest. At an average heart rate of 70 beats per minute, the human heart beats 4,200 times an hour, 100,800 times a day, 37 million times a year, and an amazing 3 billion times over an 85-year lifetime. The heart pump is divided into two halves, right and left, separated by a muscular wall called the *septum*. Each half has two chambers, the upper *atrium* and the lower *ventricle*. Blood flows into the right atrium and then, through a valve, into the right ventricle. When the right ventricle is full, another valve opens and the heart contracts, or pumps. This sends the blood from the right ventricle to the lungs, where it picks up oxygen. Oxygenated blood returning from the lungs enters the left atrium, then the left ventricle. When the valve between these two chambers closes, the heart contracts again and pumps blood into the arteries, the network of "pipes" that delivers oxygenated blood to your body.

The Pipes

Your blood vessels—the pipes—are pretty amazing, too. This complex network of tubular passageways carries blood from the heart to tissues throughout the body and back again to the heart. Freshly oxygenated blood leaving the heart enters the aorta, the large artery connected to the left ventricle, which branches off into large, elastic arteries and smaller *arterioles*. Your vascular system contains more than 100,000 arterioles, many of which are less than ⅟₁₀₀ inch in diameter. Arteries have thick, elastic walls made of smooth muscle tissue that allows them to expand and contract in response to changes in pressure against them caused by the heart's rhythmic pumping action. As the muscular arteries contract and relax, they act much like reservoirs and auxiliary pumps, keeping the blood flowing during the resting phase of the heartbeat.

Arterioles are the smallest of the arteries. They deliver oxygenated blood to *capillaries* and interconnecting branchlike *capillary beds*. These tiny vessels, sometimes collectively called the *microvasculature*, are extremely thin-walled and fragile. As fluids diffuse through the capillary walls, nutrients, gases, hormones, and other vital components are delivered to the tissues, and waste products of cellular metabolism are picked up.

The blood then begins its journey back to the heart, flowing from capillaries into small *venules* that merge to form larger veins. Veins have thinner, less muscular walls than arteries, but their diameter is wider and they are equipped with a complex series of valves. Unlike the blood flow through the arteries, which is assisted by the muscles in the vessels themselves, venous blood flow is assisted by pressure changes that occur when you breathe, which suck blood upward. This is known as the *respiratory pump*. In addition, as the skeletal muscles throughout your body contract and relax, they move venous blood toward the heart, a phenomenon called the *muscular pump*. (This explains why your feet and ankles swell when you sit or stand for long periods of time. The muscles in your lower extremities are not active enough to help move blood up through the veins, resulting in pooling of blood and swelling.) All the while, the valves in the veins prevent backflow.

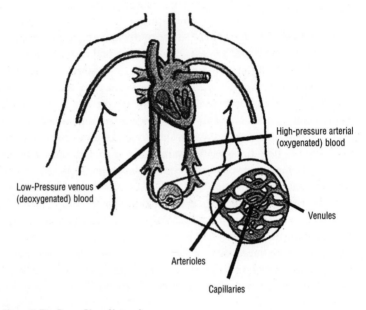

Figure 3. The Pump-Pipes Network

The Fluid

I want to say just a few words about the fluid this pump-and-pipes system circulates. Blood is the river of life. It carries all the things essential for life that must be delivered from one part of your body to another, such as oxygen, glucose, essential fats, proteins, vitamins, minerals, and hormones. It is also responsible for moving out waste products of cellular metabolism for elimination from the body. In addition, blood helps regulate body temperature, pH (acid-base balance), and fluid volume within the circulatory system. The entire purpose of the complex and elegant cardiovascular system is the transportation of life-sustaining blood throughout the body.

PUMP, PIPES, AND BLOOD PRESSURE

Now let's see how blood pressure fits in. In any enclosed pump-and-pipes system, the pump creates fluid flow, and pressure results as the fluid flowing through the pipes encounters resistance, or friction. Every beat of your heart generates a powerful thrust that pumps blood through the pipes of the vascular system, creating pressure in the vessels. Each time the heart relaxes between beats, the pressure in the system falls temporarily, while the pump chambers refill with blood. When the chambers are full, the heart pumps blood through the pipes once again. In hydraulics, this is described as "pulsatile flow," meaning that the fluid flows in waves, or pulsations, and it's why blood pressure is described with two numbers. Systolic pressure, the top and larger number in the ratio, is the peak pressure of the fluid in the pipes (arteries) just after the heart has pumped. The diastolic pressure, the bottom and smaller number, refers to the pressure in the pipes between pumps, when the heart is at rest.

Blood pressure is highest in the arteries and arterioles and lowest in the capillaries and veins. Blood oozes from a cut vein, but it spurts from a lacerated artery. This reflects the significant pressure differences between arteries and veins, and it also explains why arteries are the blood vessels most affected by hypertension. Blood pressure is highest of all in the arteries nearest the aorta, the main artery just off the heart. The pressure there is so great that if the aorta itself were lacerated, blood would squirt out five or six feet!

The farther the arteries are from the heart, the lower the pressure becomes, until it reaches the arterioles. The small size of the arterioles creates natural resistance to the blood flowing from the larger arteries. As a result, pressure goes up in the arteries—and up even more when the arterioles constrict. The blood then moves into the capillaries and capillary beds. Blood pressure is necessarily low on these tiny, thin-walled, fragile vessels. Blood leaving the capillaries and entering the venules and veins remains under low pressure—too low, in fact, for the blood to return to the heart without some help. Therefore, blood flow in the venous system is assisted by the respiratory and muscular pumps and the venous valves, as described above.

The pressure in any pump-pipes system can shift with changes in any one or a combination of three things: pumping intensity, rate, and output; fluid volume of the system; and resistance on the pipes. Here's how these factors correspond to the pressure of blood in your own pump-and-pipes system.

- *Pumping intensity, rate, and output.* The more intense or rapid the heartbeat, the greater the volume of blood pumped out of the heart with each beat (known as *cardiac output*) and the higher the blood pressure throughout the system. Stress or exercise, for example, prompts the adrenal glands to secrete hormones that speed up heart rate and cardiac output. This in turn elevates blood pressure.
- *Fluid volume.* The more blood in the system, the greater the pressure against the blood vessel walls. Blood volume increases—and blood pressure rises—when sodium levels increase and cause water to be retained by the body. This results from dietary indiscretions and mineral imbalances.
- *Resistance on the pipes.* As blood flows through the vessels, it encounters friction or a phenomenon known as *peripheral resistance* (because the greatest friction is in the peripheral arterioles, away from the heart). Three things contribute to peripheral resistance. One is blood viscosity, or thickness. The thicker the blood, the less easily it flows and the higher the blood pressure. Excess fat in the diet may contribute to increased blood viscosity. Another contributor to peripheral resistance is total blood vessel length—the longer the length, the greater the resistance. Every extra pound on your body requires additional blood vessels to sustain it, and this is one reason why weight gain is associated with increases in blood pressure.

  The third and perhaps most significant cause of peripheral resistance and increased blood pressure is decreased diameter and responsiveness of the arteries and arterioles. The muscular walls of your arteries and arterioles enable them to constrict and expand to divert blood to various areas, depending on your body's needs. When they constrict and become smaller—decreasing the diameter of the pipes—blood pressure goes up. The arteries and arterioles constrict in response to hormones and other chemical messengers associated with stress, exercise, and other factors, as well as to mineral imbalances at the cellular level. In addition, *arteriosclerosis* (stiffening and thickening of the arteries) and *atherosclerosis* (buildup of plaque in the arteries) also decrease the diameter and flexibility of the arteries, thus contributing to peripheral resistance and higher blood pressure.

BLOOD PRESSURE: THE REST OF THE STORY

Maintaining steady blood flow to all of the organs of your body is essential, and it requires constant adjustments by your cardiovascular system. When you're walking or running, for example, more blood than usual is required in your legs, so your heart rate and cardiac output go up. The arteries leading to the legs dilate and their capillary beds open, delivering more blood to the working muscles. When you eat, the arteries leading to the stomach and intestines dilate in a similar manner, providing additional blood needed for digestion and nutrient absorption. Likewise, when you jump out of bed in the morning, the heart must work harder and blood pressure must increase to deliver blood and oxygen to the brain. Throughout the day and night, your arteries continuously guide the rivers of blood to where they're needed most. And constant automatic adjustments in your blood pressure, which require the coordination of your nervous system, endocrine system, and kidneys, are made all the while.

▼ | NITRIC OXIDE: THE MISSING LINK?

Nitric oxide is a molecule derived from the amino acid arginine that has been discovered in recent years to have myriad functions in the human body. More than 10,000 articles have been published in peer-reviewed medical journals in the past ten years on nitric oxide, which acts as a neurotransmitter in the brain, a targeted chemical in the immune system, and a messenger molecule throughout the body. Altered nitric oxide function has been implicated in diseases ranging from cancer to AIDS to heart disease and hypertension.

Nitric oxide is released by the endothelial cells lining the arteries and arterioles. Although its effects are short-lived, nitric oxide is one of the most powerful vasodilators known. By relaxing the smooth muscles and thus increasing the diameter of the blood vessels, nitric oxide is a principal regulator of blood pressure. It is also a player in atherosclerosis, the stiffening and narrowing of arterial walls, as it protects the arteries by preventing the adhesion of platelets and white blood cells. Conversely, arteries that have been damaged by atherosclerosis have impaired synthesis of nitric oxide. In addition, nitric oxide has powerful antioxidant activity. Therefore, this substance plays multiple roles in hypertension.

The Nervous and Endocrine Systems

Changes in blood pressure are orchestrated by the nervous system. *Baroreceptors*, specialized receptors in the aorta and arteries of the neck and thorax, send messages to the brain when modifications in blood pressure need to be made. This in turn signals changes in the rate and force of the contractions of the heart and in the diameter of the blood vessels. The vasomotor center located in the brain stem, the oldest area of your brain and the part that is responsible for the most basic needs of life, controls blood pressure. But other centers in the brain play a role as well, particularly when stress is involved.

You probably know from personal experience that your blood pressure rises during periods of stress. When you are scared or anxious or feel threatened in any way, your body automatically kicks into what is called the *stress response*. The stress response is a natural survival tool and a carryover from the days when most of the threats humans faced were physical. Meeting up with a hostile, club-wielding tribe or a saber-tooth tiger required a "fight-or-flight" response, and our bodies immediately readied for action. Although few of our modern stressors—traffic jams, deadlines, disagreements with coworkers or family members, and the like—can be solved by running away or duking it out, our bodies nevertheless respond in the same manner.

During the stress response an area of the brain called the *hypothalamus* signals the pituitary gland to release a hormone that activates the adrenal glands. The adrenal churns out the stress hormones *epinephrine* (also called *adrenaline*) and *norepinephrine* (or noradrenaline). These chemical messengers stimulate beta and alpha receptors in the heart and blood vessels. Your heart rate becomes faster and more intense, and blood vessels constrict to direct blood to your muscles, so you'll be able to run faster and fight harder. Digestion slows down as blood is transported away from the stomach, and you receive an extra burst of blood sugar for additional energy. Your brain and senses are alert and responsive. This is an automatic response, carried out by the autonomic nervous system, which manages your body's involuntary functions. But it also temporarily raises blood pressure by increasing cardiac output and resistance on the blood vessels. So you can see how repeated stress contributes to consistently elevated blood pressure. Chronic stress is very damaging to systems throughout your body. Over time, it depletes your body of magnesium, potassium, and other essential nutrients, which further contributes to hypertension. (In Chapter 14, I will give you valuable tools to combat daily stress.)

The Kidneys

The kidneys also play an important role in blood pressure control. Their primary function is to purify the blood and regulate its composition—they filter out impurities and return important blood components to circulation. These busy organs, which are located at the back of the abdominal cavity on either side of the spine, filter gallons of blood every hour. The kidneys operate through a highly developed duct system of more than a million funnels called *nephrons*. Functioning much like checkpoints or monitoring stations, nephrons determine whether substances should be directed back into the blood or excreted. The kidneys constantly monitor and adjust sodium levels, which determine the amount of fluid circulating in the system. In this way, the kidneys function as a blood volume—and blood pressure—control valve.

▼ HORMONES AND OTHER CHEMICAL MESSENGERS THAT AFFECT BLOOD PRESSURE

Epinephrine and norepinephrine	Released by the adrenal glands in response to stress; increase cardiac output and constrict arterioles
Aldosterone	Released by the adrenal glands as prompted by angiotensin II; causes salt and water retention
Antidiuretic hormone (ADH)	Produced by the hypothalamus when blood pressure is very low; causes salt and water retention and constricts the arterioles
Angiotensin II	Generated by the RAAS (described below); constricts arterioles and stimulates release of ADH and aldosterone
Nitric oxide	Released by the lining of the arteries; relaxes blood vessels and improves blood flow

The Renin-Angiotensin-Aldosterone System

One of the most important determinants of blood pressure is the *renin-angiotensin-aldosterone system* (RAAS), which is named for three of the compounds involved in this complex series of biochemical reactions. Although the RAAS plays a role in daily fluctuations in blood pressure, it is also a key player in longer-term regulation, and in hypertension.

Here's how the RAAS system works. *Angiotensinogen* is a protein produced in the liver on a continuous basis. *Renin* is an enzyme that is released by the kidneys under conditions of stress, exercise, or certain changes in diet. When angiotensinogen and renin join in the bloodstream, they form *angiotensin I*. As the blood carrying angiotensin I travels through the lungs, it reacts with *angiotensin-converting enzyme* (ACE) to form *angiotensin II*. Angiotensin II has two actions. First, it causes the muscular walls of the arteries, and particularly the arterioles, to contract. This decreases their diameter and drives up blood pressure. Second, angiotensin II prompts the adrenal glands (located on top of the kidneys) to release *aldosterone*. Aldosterone is a hormone that signals the kidneys to keep more sodium and water in the bloodstream and stop excreting them through the urine. This results in increased blood volume and higher blood pressure. (It also explains why excess salt in the diet raises blood pressure, as we will discuss in Chapter 8.)

The RAAS is crucial for your health and well-being. Remember, the diameter of your blood vessels and your blood pressure are in constant flux as the needs of your body change from moment to moment, and this is one of the mechanisms that oversees these normal variations. However, when the RAAS pathway becomes overactive, blood pressure is consistently elevated. This is estimated to be the primary cause of high blood pressure in about a third of all people with hypertension.

TWO TYPES OF HYPERTENSION

There are two types of hypertension. The most common type is *primary hypertension*, sometimes referred to as *essential hypertension*. (This term was coined in the early 1800s by English physician Richard Bright, and it refers to the prevailing theory of the time that high blood pressure was an essential response of the body to ensure blood flow to the vital organs.) Up to 95 percent of all patients with hypertension have this type, which is attributed to and may be modified by diet, exercise, and other lifestyle habits. However, 5 to 10 percent of those with hypertension have *secondary hypertension*, in which high blood pressure stems from an underlying physical cause, such as kidney disease or adrenal disorders. Although secondary hypertension is rare, if you have high blood pressure, this condition needs to be ruled out.

COMMON CAUSES OF SECONDARY HYPERTENSION

- Chronic renal (kidney) disease, renal artery stenosis, or renal vascular arteriosclerosis
- Adrenal disorders, such as tumors, excessive production of aldosterone, or Cushing's syndrome
- Congenital defect of the aorta
- History of cocaine or other substance abuse

If, for example, a tumor is pressing on specialized tissue of the adrenal glands called chromaffin tissue, the excess pressure will provoke the glands to produce abnormally high levels of the hormones epinephrine and norepinephrine. These chemical messengers cause the heart to pump harder and the blood pressure to rise. Removal of the tumor will relieve the pressure on the chromaffin tissue and thereby normalize hormone production and blood pressure.

One of my patients, Elizabeth, was suffering from a number of health complaints, including hypertension. None of her doctors could understand why her blood pressure fluctuated so dramatically until one physician found an obstruction in the renal artery, leading to her kidney. The blockage caused her kidney to perceive the blood pressure as being low—which it was on the kidney side of the blockage. This false perception caused her kidneys to compensate by releasing renin, which, as described above, activates the RAAS pathway to constrict the arteries and cause blood pressure to go up. When the blockage was removed, Elizabeth's kidneys were able to determine her true blood pressure and normalize renin production. She now reports having lower and more consistent blood pressure, which indicates that her hypertension was secondary to an underlying medical condition.

It can sometimes be tricky to diagnose secondary hypertension. Researchers Robert J. Heyka, M.D., and Donald G. Vidt, M.D., at the Cleveland Clinic Foundation, devised a four-point checklist that helps doctors narrow the possibilities of secondary hypertension. If you have hypertension and any of these apply to you, make sure to let your physician know right away.

- The sudden onset of high blood pressure
- Hypertension developed before age 30 or after age 55
- Hypertension previously controlled through medication but now high, or on the sudden rise
- Stage 3 hypertension (systolic higher than 180 mm Hg or diastolic higher than 110 mm Hg)

Secondary hypertension is serious business, but its underlying causes can often be corrected. Don't forget, however, that it accounts for only 5 to 10 percent of all cases of hypertension. The vast majority of patients with high blood pressure have primary hypertension, which can be addressed through the program for reversing hypertension described in Part II of this book.

CHAPTER 3

Heart Attacks, Strokes, and Other Hazards of Hypertension

Betty was a vivacious, healthy 58-year-old with no apparent medical problems. She worked alongside her husband running their farm, and her workload and stamina would put most of us to shame. Betty was one of those people who rarely get sick—even when a cold or flu swept through the house she never seemed to catch it. She hadn't seen a doctor since the birth of her youngest child. She just couldn't see the need for it.

One day without warning Betty suddenly began to feel weak and confused. The left side of her body felt numb, and she had difficulty speaking. Betty had suffered a stroke—the first sign that she had hypertension.

Hypertension is stealthy. Like Betty, one-third of all patients with high blood pressure are unaware that they have any problem at all. Unlike the aches and pains that accompany arthritis, or the chronic cough that signals a respiratory disorder, warning signs of hypertension may be subtle or nonexistent for many years. Yet all the while your blood vessels, heart, and other organ systems are taking a silent beating. Your heart becomes overworked and begins to falter. Your blood vessels wear down under the relentless pounding they are subjected to and are further damaged by atherosclerosis. As blood flow to your organs becomes inadequate, your heart, kidneys, brain, and nervous system all suffer serious damage.

▼ │ HAZARDS OF HYPERTENSION

- Triples risk of dying from a *heart attack*
- Quadruples risk of *heart failure*
- Increases risk of dying from *stroke* sevenfold
- Increases risk of *dementia* and *Alzheimer's disease*
- Intensifies aging process in kidneys (second leading cause of *chronic kidney failure*)
- Accelerates damage to arteries, leading to *atherosclerosis* and *arteriosclerosis*

HYPERTENSION WEARS OUT THE HEART

According to the American Heart Association, hypertension is a contributing factor in the 1.1 million heart attacks and more than 300,000 heart attack deaths in the United States each year. Hypertension hurts the heart by pushing it to the limits. Years of overexertion cause the heart to become weak and damaged—the pump just wears out.

Hypertension is the leading risk factor for heart attack, or myocardial infarction (MI). A heart attack occurs when part of the heart's blood supply is suddenly reduced or cut off, usually due to a blockage in one of the coronary arteries supplying blood to the heart. The portions of the heart muscle that cannot get adequate oxygen and nutrients die. The more extensive the damage, the more serious the heart attack.

Hypertension is also the chief cause of *left ventricular hypertrophy*, one of the hallmarks of hypertension, especially untreated hypertension. Like any muscle, the heart bulks up with overuse. In particular, the muscular walls of the left ventricle—the discharge chamber that actually pumps blood into the arterial system—thicken and swell. As the walls thicken, the volume of the chamber shrinks, and the amount of blood it can hold and pump throughout the body is reduced. Because the heart is now pumping less blood with each beat, it works even harder to maintain circulation. This may lead to further weakening of the heart—it simply tires out and swells up like a weak balloon. This end-stage disease is called *congestive heart failure* (CHF). The pumping efficiency of the heart is now so poor that it cannot maintain adequate circulation of the blood. Blood pools in the vessels and the patient becomes weak and has difficulty breathing. The swollen, hypertrophied heart muscle becomes so overburdened that it eventually just stops working.

▼ HYPERTENSION PREMATURELY AGES THE BLOOD VESSELS

You probably know someone whose appearance belies their age. It might be their dry, wrinkled skin or slow, shuffling gait, but they appear older than their years. Well, blood vessels are also subject to premature aging. As we age, changes in the *endothelium* (the lining of the blood vessels) occur that result in a gradual stiffening and loss of elasticity. The blood vessels become less responsive to blood-borne chemical messengers and are unable to relax normally, decreasing their ability to deliver blood where it is needed most. This may result in stroke, heart attack, or one of the other hazards of hypertension discussed in this chapter.

According to a report from the American Heart Association, "This process fast-forwards in people with high blood pressure, causing their blood vessels to age prematurely." Dr. Walter Kirkendall, professor of medicine and director of the Hypertension Unit, University of Texas Medical School in Houston, takes it a step further and states, "Vascular disease caused by hypertension intensifies the aging processes in the kidney, brain, and heart."

TOP RISK FACTOR FOR STROKE

Stroke is the third leading cause of death in America, and for many people, like Betty, a stroke comes out of the blue, with little or no warning. Hypertension is the primary factor underlying the 731,000 strokes and 160,000 stroke-related deaths that occur annually. Too much pressure can cause the bursting of a vessel—especially if that vessel has been weakened by age and the excess pressure of hypertension. Hypertension also contributes to atherosclerosis and arteriosclerosis, the narrowing and stiffening of the arteries that increases the likelihood of blood clots cutting off blood supply. When either of these scenarios occurs in an artery in the brain, the result is a stroke, also called a *cerebrovascular accident* or *brain attack*. There is a reduction in oxygen supply to that area of the brain, followed by cell degeneration and death.

Stroke is the number one cause of long-term disability in America. Roughly 80 percent of stroke survivors will end up physically impaired, with about 40 percent suffering mild physical disability and the remaining 40 percent becoming severely disabled. There are more than 4 million stroke survivors alive today, many of whom are disabled, and we can expect over half a million new stroke victims this year.

HYPERTENSION AND YOUR BRAIN

A lesser-known outcome of hypertension is memory loss and an increased risk of dementia and Alzheimer's disease. The adverse effects of hypertension on mental functioning have been verified in several large-scale studies. One of these studies, the 1995 Honolulu-Asia Aging Study, was based on the evaluation of 3,735 Japanese-American men living in Hawaii. Researchers compared these men's midlife blood pressures to their late-life cognitive function. They discovered that elevated systolic blood pressure in midlife was a significant predictor of diminished mental function in later life.

Another study, published in *The Lancet* in 1996, found similar relationships between elevated blood pressure in older people and the development of Alzheimer's disease. In this study, 382 Swedes were followed for fifteen years. Researchers found that the study subjects who had hypertension at age 70 also had an increased risk of developing dementia by age 85. When compared with those who had no mental deficits, patients who developed Alzheimer's between the ages of 79 and 95 were more likely to have had an elevated diastolic reading at age 70. In addition, those with a higher diastolic reading at age 75 were much more likely to develop dementia between the ages of 79 and 85.

It is believed that hypertension's adverse effects on the brain are caused by the relentless pounding on the small vessels in the brain. The brains of patients with high blood pressure actually shrink—by as much as 20 percent, according to some studies. Although other studies estimate the shrinkage to be much smaller, researchers point out that even minute changes in important structures of the brain may have serious consequences. A long-term study sponsored by the National Heart, Lung, and Blood Institute, which has followed more than 1,000 men for over thirty years, supports this. Early results of this study show that men in their seventies who had hypertension in their forties not only had smaller brains than their healthy peers, but also other changes associated with premature aging of the brain.

Another reason hypertension hastens mental deterioration is that it dramatically increases stroke risk. It has recently been discovered that repeated small strokes—which are often so minor they are not even noticed—are a significant risk factor for Alzheimer's disease. Among the first to observe this was Dr. David Snowdon, of the University of Kentucky Sanders-Brown Center on Aging, who is spearheading an ongoing study on mental function and aging. For several years now, Dr. Snowdon and his colleagues have followed nuns living in a convent in Mankato, Minnesota, focusing primarily on their mental function as they age. A 1997 report coming out of the "Nun Study," based on the autopsies of 102 nuns, found that small strokes, including "silent" strokes, were an important contributor to the development of Alzheimer's disease.

HIGH BLOOD PRESSURE INCREASES RISK OF KIDNEY DISEASE

Hypertension also accelerates the aging of the kidneys. High blood pressure damages the arteries and arterioles that supply blood and nutrients to the kidneys. As these arteries become stiff and less elastic, blood supply to the kidneys is reduced or, in some cases, cut off, causing damage to the kidneys themselves. This condition, known as *hypertensive nephrosclerosis*, is a significant cause of kidney malfunction. Severe high blood pressure causes kidney malfunction over a relatively short period of time; however, even milder forms of uncontrolled hypertension can damage kidneys over several years, with no evident symptoms until severe damage has already occurred. Poorly controlled high blood pressure is responsible for approximately 25 percent of all cases of chronic kidney failure. Hypertension is also second only to diabetes as the leading cause of end-stage renal disease, which necessitates dialysis or kidney transplantation.

ATHEROSCLEROSIS AND ARTERIOSCLEROSIS: CAUSES OR RESULTS OF HYPERTENSION?

Atherosclerosis is the deposition of fat and cholesterol (plaque build-up) in the artery walls, which causes them to thicken and their diameter to narrow. As plaque formation interferes with the absorption of nutrients by the arteries, they sustain further damage. Smooth muscle cells die, arteries lose their elasticity and become rigid and unresponsive, and artery walls begin to ulcerate and become jagged and frayed. The end stage of this process is arteriosclerosis. These two terms, atherosclerosis and arteriosclerosis, are often used interchangeably. Atherosclerosis is the more popular term, so we'll use it here. But whatever you call it, it dramatically increases the risk of heart attack, stroke, and circulatory problems.

As atherosclerosis progresses, the ability of the endothelial cells lining the arteries to release nitric oxide and other chemicals that relax the vessels and lower blood pressure is impaired. To make matters worse, scar tissue forms in the arteries and they become hard and stiff. This destructive process may eventually block blood vessels, cut off blood flow, and set you up for a stroke or heart attack.

Although researchers have long associated hypertension with the increased risk of atherosclerosis, they can't seem to agree on which comes first. Hypertension appears to be both a major cause *and* a result of atherosclerosis. Although high blood pressure may initiate and definitely exacerbates atherosclerosis, this condition may precede hypertension—and the resulting narrowed arteries (decreased pipe diameter) increase blood pressure. In addition, as the narrowed, stiffened arteries become less responsive to nerve impulses, hormones, and other messenger chemicals, they simply fail to respond to the body's internal blood pressure regulation systems.

Now that you realize the extent of damage associated with high blood pressure, let's take a look at the role we ourselves have played in bringing on this condition.

CHAPTER 4

The Primary Causes of Hypertension

When Rick was in the army during the Korean War, he was told that he had high blood pressure. However, he wasn't offered any treatment, and since he had no symptoms—after all, he was in his invincible twenties at the time—he pretty much ignored it. After his discharge Rick got a job with the transit system in Cleveland, Ohio, where he worked for the next forty years. Rick was a hard worker, and he rose in the ranks to become an officer of his union local. This was an extremely stressful position, and among the things that helped Rick cope were heavy drinking and chain smoking. As time went by, Rick's blood pressure became sky-high.

Any physician worth his salt would know that Rick was heading for trouble. He perfectly fit the profile of a patient at risk for developing hypertension. Yet the American Heart Association continues to maintain that in 90 to 95 percent of all cases of high blood pressure, the cause is unknown. Hogwash! In truth, hypertension is primarily a disease of lifestyle, caused by poor nutrition, obesity, inactivity, smoking, heavy drinking, and chronic stress. These lifestyle habits interfere with the self-regulating mechanisms that keep blood pressure under control. They accelerate the aging of the cardiovascular system, causing it to give out before its time. While some of the causes of hypertension are outside your control, the important message of this chapter is that you *do* have control over the most significant risk factors for high blood pressure.

CONTROLLABLE RISK FACTORS FOR HYPERTENSION

- Obesity
- Insulin resistance and type II diabetes
- High-fat/cholesterol diet
- Diet high in sugar and refined carbohydrates
- High-salt diet
- Low-potassium diet
- Nutritional deficiencies (potassium, magnesium, calcium, antioxidants, and B-complex vitamins)
- Smoking
- Heavy drinking
- Chronic stress

OBESITY AND HYPERTENSION GO HAND IN HAND

Obesity, defined as being 20 percent above your ideal body weight, is the single most significant factor related to hypertension. Among the obese, hypertension is three times more common than it is in those of normal weight. A gender breakdown of these statistics shows that in 78 percent of men with hypertension and 65 percent of women, the condition is directly related to obesity. It's no wonder then that hypertension rates are soaring in this country. We are in the midst of an epidemic of obesity. According to former U.S. Surgeon General C. Everett Koop, M.D., in a 1998 letter to the *Wall Street Journal,*

In sheer numbers and its costs to society, obesity has reached crisis proportions in the U.S. Whether one calls it a "disease" or simply a "condition," the facts remain the same: obesity has increased at record levels over the past decade, up from 26 percent of adults in 1980 to 34 percent today. As a result, over 58 million American adults—one third of the population—are overweight or obese. At the same time, childhood obesity rates have been rising steadily over the last three decades, with 22 percent of children ages 6 to 17 now overweight. . . . Obesity is directly linked to a number of disabling and life-threatening diseases—diabetes, hypertension, heart disease, some forms of cancer, gallbladder disease, and osteoarthritis—which will continue to adversely affect the lives of many Americans.

Obesity and hypertension go hand in hand for several reasons. One has to do with peripheral resistance, or friction on the "pipes," which, as we discussed in Chapter 2, is one of the variables that increase blood pressure. The more body fat you carry, the more blood vessels and capillaries you must have to feed this extra tissue. One factor that increases resistance on the pipes, or blood vessels, is their total length—the longer the vessels, the more resistance blood flow encounters. According to Elaine Marieb, R.N., Ph.D., author of *Human Anatomy & Physiology*, every extra pound or two of fat requires the addition of literally miles of vessels to service it. This significantly increases peripheral resistance and contributes to the elevation of blood pressure in obese people.

Another link between obesity and hypertension hinges on a condition called *insulin resistance*, in which cells are unable to properly respond to insulin. Insulin resistance is an underlying condition in about half of all people with hypertension. It also is strongly associated with abnormalities in blood sugar and blood fats, increased risk of diabetes and heart disease, and obesity. The type of obesity associated with insulin resistance is quite specific. Fat storage in the thighs and buttocks does not pose a problem or increase the risk of the medical problems associated with insulin resistance. This type of fat distribution is commonly referred to as "pear-shaped obesity" in contrast to the more ominous "apple-shaped obesity." People with an apple shape carry excess weight around their middle—the old spare tire, potbelly, or beer gut. Apple-shaped obesity, also called central obesity or abdominal obesity, is a hallmark of insulin resistance and may increase the risk of heart disease, diabetes, and other serious medical conditions. (More on this in Chapter 6.)

Numerous studies reveal that a simple reduction of body fat is often enough to reduce blood pressure to healthier levels. One study demonstrating this link was published in the *Archives of Internal Medicine*. In this study, 301 obese patients with hypertension were enrolled in a weight loss program, consisting of behavior modification, medication, or a combination of the two. Weight loss in these patients was associated with significant reductions in systolic and diastolic blood pressure. The 36 patients in the study who did not lose weight had no decrease in blood pressure.

Researchers at Mount Sinai Medical Center in New York, recognizing that ideal body weight is difficult to achieve, have found that even losing 10 pounds may help control blood pressure. These and other studies with similar outcomes are a testament to the power of diet. Achieving as close to your ideal body weight as possible should be among your top priorities as you strive to reverse hypertension. The dietary guidelines I recommend in Part II for reducing blood pressure will naturally reduce your waistline as well.

The body mass index (BMI) is a standard measure of the ratio of lean muscle mass to body fat. Figure 4 shows how BMIs (numbers in

Weight

Height	100	105	110	115	120	125	130	135	140	145	150	155	160	165	170	175	180	185	190	195	200	205
5'0"	20	21	21	22	23	24	25	26	27	28	29	30	31	32	33	34	35	36	37	38	39	40
5'1"	19	20	21	22	23	24	25	26	26	27	28	29	30	31	32	33	34	35	36	37	38	39
5'2"	18	19	20	21	22	23	24	25	26	27	27	28	29	30	31	32	33	34	35	36	37	37
5'3"	18	19	19	20	21	22	23	24	25	26	27	27	28	29	30	31	32	33	34	35	35	36
5'4"	17	18	19	20	21	21	22	23	24	25	26	27	27	28	29	30	31	32	33	33	34	35
5'5"	17	17	18	19	20	21	22	22	23	24	25	26	27	27	28	29	30	31	32	32	33	34
5'6"	16	17	18	19	19	20	21	22	23	23	24	25	26	27	27	28	29	30	31	31	32	33
5'7"	16	16	17	18	19	20	20	21	22	23	23	24	25	26	27	27	28	29	30	31	31	32
5'8"	15	16	17	17	18	19	20	21	21	22	23	24	24	25	26	27	27	28	29	30	30	31
5'9"	15	16	16	17	18	18	19	20	21	21	22	23	24	24	25	26	27	27	28	29	30	30
5'10"	14	15	16	17	17	18	19	19	20	21	22	22	23	24	24	25	26	27	27	28	29	29
5'11"	14	15	15	16	17	17	18	19	20	20	21	22	22	23	24	24	25	26	26	27	28	29
6'0"	14	14	15	16	16	17	18	18	19	20	20	21	22	22	23	24	24	25	26	26	27	28
6'1"	13	14	15	15	16	16	17	18	18	19	20	20	21	22	22	23	24	24	25	26	26	27
6'2"	13	13	14	15	15	16	17	17	18	19	19	20	21	21	22	22	23	24	24	25	26	26
6'3"	12	13	14	14	15	16	16	17	17	18	19	19	20	21	21	22	22	23	24	24	25	26
6'4"	12	13	13	14	15	15	16	16	17	18	18	19	19	20	21	21	22	23	23	24	24	25

Figure 4. Body Mass Index (BMI)

Reprinted with permission from Wickelgren I. Obesity: how big a problem? *Science*. May 29, 1998; 280(5368):1364-1367. Copyright 1998 American Association for the Advancement of Science. Source: Shape Up America.

squares) vary with weight and height. A BMI of 19 to 25 is in the healthy range; a BMI of 26 and above, however, puts you at increased risk for several degenerative diseases, including hypertension.

DIETARY FACTORS CONTRIBUTING TO HYPERTENSION

The modern American diet is without precedent. Never before in human history has any culture consumed so much unnatural food. There is a lot of controversy today over the type of diet humans have evolved to eat. Are we meat-eating hunters or plant-consuming gatherers? Based on the human tooth structure and intestinal tract, as well as observations of surviving Stone Age tribes of hunters and gatherers, we're probably meant to be vegetarians and "opportunistic" meat eaters. What we are not designed to eat—and there is no controversy on this point—is the array of fatty, salty, refined, processed foods, stripped of fiber and nutrients, that make up the bulk of the American diet. And we are paying the price for these poor eating habits with obesity, hypertension, heart disease, cancer, and a host of other degenerative diseases. A diet rich in animal fats, sugar, refined carbohydrates, and salt—and deficient in plant foods that contain an abundance of antioxidants, minerals, and other nutrients—is a significant contributor to the American epidemic of degenerative diseases. And obesity and high blood pressure are near the top of this list.

High-Fat Diet

Volumes of scientific literature support the negative impact of a high-fat diet on the cardiovascular system. A high-fat diet contributes to obesity, which increases peripheral resistance in the arterioles and can drive blood pressure up. It is a proven factor in atherosclerosis, which narrows the "pipes." Fat also interferes with insulin utilization and contributes to insulin resistance, which is a significant factor in many cases of hypertension (Chapter 6 is devoted to this subject).

Dr. Salah Kassab, of the University of Mississippi Medical Center in Jackson, suggests that a high-fat diet also results in sodium retention, which increases blood volume and drives up blood pressure. This was demonstrated in an experiment in which dogs were fed a high-fat diet for a period of five weeks. Not only did the dogs gain an average of 8 pounds, but their blood pressure and heart rate also rose considerably. By the end of the study, their diastolic blood pressure soared from 87 to 91 mm Hg, and the resting heart rate increased a whopping 20 beats per minute (from 83 to 113).

The kind of fat you eat makes a difference, too. Fats that contribute to heart disease include cholesterol-laden saturated fats from meat, eggs and high-fat dairy products, and overly processed vegetable oils. When polyunsaturated vegetable oils are processed under high temperatures, they may transmute into unnatural breakdown products that are harmful to the arteries. Margarine and solid vegetable shortening are particularly dangerous as their processing results in the formation of toxic *trans fatty acids*. These altered fats—which are like nothing Mother Nature ever intended—interfere with some of your body's important functions. In Part II you'll learn about beneficial fats that actually help reverse hypertension.

Sugar and Refined Carbohydrates

A diet high in sugar and refined carbohydrates contributes to hypertension in a number of ways. First, such a diet promotes obesity. In the past few years, fat has been singled out as public enemy number one, and we've become virtual fat phobics. However, in place of fatty foods, we have turned to carbohydrates—in any shape or form. Statistics show that this hasn't put a dent in the problem of obesity. In fact, it's gotten worse, as the ranks of the obese have swelled from 25 percent to 33 percent of all Americans.

Second, excess intake of sugar and other simple carbohydrates as a factor in and of itself also increases blood pressure. A diet high in processed and refined carbohydrates—one in which these foods contribute 50 to 80 percent of total daily calories—has been demonstrated to promote sodium retention, which, as we have noted, increases blood volume and in turn raises blood pressure. Third, in the last ten years scientists have discovered new relationships between dietary sugar and refined carbohydrates and diseases such as hypertension, diabetes, and heart disease.

▼ DOES COFFEE RAISE BLOOD PRESSURE?

Cappuccino, latte, mocha, anyone? A cup or two of coffee is a harmless way to start out your day—or is it? The relationship between caffeine and blood pressure has been evaluated in hundreds of scientific studies over the past few decades. And although the bulk of these studies provide no solid evidence that moderate caffeine consumption significantly raises blood pressure over the long run, caffeine does at least temporarily affect blood pressure.

Dr. James Lane and colleagues at Duke University assessed the effects of caffeine on 72 coffee drinkers in a two-week study conducted in 1999. The men and women in this study were given 250 milligrams of caffeine (the equivalent of about two to two and a half 6-ounce cups of coffee) in capsule form at eight o'clock in the morning and another 250 milligrams at noon during the first week of the study. They were given capsules containing an inert substance (*placebo*) on a similar schedule during the second week, while abstaining from other caffeine sources. There was a dramatic increase in stress hormone levels and a 2 mm Hg increase in systolic and diastolic blood pressures in the subjects when they were taking caffeine, compared to when they were taking a placebo. Furthermore, blood pressure remained slightly elevated throughout the day, until ten o'clock in the evening. Even this small increase can adversely affect your health. According to Dr. Lane, "A 5 mm Hg increase in blood pressure is associated with a 34 percent increase in incidence of stroke and a 21 percent increase in incidence of heart disease."

If you feel it's important that you have a cup of coffee in the morning, have one small cup. (A 6-ounce cup of coffee contains 90–120 milligrams of caffeine, depending on the method of preparation.) But don't drink it all day. Or better yet, give it up altogether.

Excess Salt

Because of its chemical structure, sodium circulating in the bloodstream forces water to follow it. It's part of a beautifully designed system that maintains fluid balance and facilitates the absorption of nutrients into the bloodstream to be delivered throughout your body. However, excess salt (sodium chloride) in the diet causes too much sodium to be dumped into the bloodstream, which may result in increased water and blood volume. And increased blood volume, as you recall from Chapter 2, is a fundamental contributor to hypertension. Interestingly, salt doesn't affect us all in the same way. While minute amounts may drive blood pressure up in individuals who are acutely sensitive to salt, other individuals may consume even larger amounts with no effect on blood pressure. Salt sensitivity appears to be an inherited phenomenon, and scientists at the University of Utah School of Medicine in Salt Lake City believe they may have actually identified a "salt gene."

Although salt has traditionally been considered the principal dietary factor in raising blood pressure, not all research supports this view. In fact, some evidence suggests that a sodium-free diet may have unfavorable effects of its own. Furthermore, some scientists have looked at the other component in table salt, chloride. Several studies have determined that it is the combination of these two minerals that drives up blood pressure in salt-sensitive individuals, not sodium alone. Two studies comparing the effects of sodium chloride and sodium citrate (another form of salt) on two groups of hypertensive patients found that blood pressure only increased in those who used sodium chloride, suggesting that chloride might be the more harmful aspect of salt. The subject of salt and blood pressure is much more complex than most people think, and Chapter 8 considers it in greater detail.

Potassium-Poor Diet

There is so much talk about sodium's role in hypertension that we often forget the other half of the equation, potassium. Minerals often work in tandem in your body: calcium and magnesium, zinc and copper, manganese and iron—and sodium and potassium. These mineral "couples" act in an interdependent fashion, and deficiencies or excesses in one will upset their delicate balance, affecting how the other is utilized and stored. The partnership of potassium and sodium is particularly strong. These two minerals work together to give your cells their important electrical charges and to help transport nutrients across cellular membranes. And because sodium and potassium are so closely intertwined, both play an important role in blood pressure.

In fact, as I will explain in Chapter 8, it is the *balance* of these two minerals, more than the level of each individually, that affects blood pressure. This is bad news for modern Americans who gorge on salty foods and avoid potassium-rich vegetables, fruits, and other plant foods. For these people the sodium-potassium balance is weighed heavily in favor of sodium, with sometimes disastrous consequences. Medical research has finally established the role of a diet abundant in potassium-containing plant foods in preventing and reversing hypertension. Some studies have gone a step further and determined that potassium supplements are useful in both the prevention and treatment of high blood pressure.

Nutritional Deficiencies

Deficiencies in other nutrients, in addition to potassium, have been linked to the development of hypertension and to insulin resistance. Foremost among these are magnesium and calcium. Recent research published in the *American Journal of Clinical Nutrition* demonstrated that when adults had adequate intakes of magnesium, calcium, and potassium, a diet high in sodium was not associated with elevated blood pressure. In fact, even in the face of a high-salt diet, individuals who got lots of other minerals through diet or nutritional supplements had the lowest blood pressure observed in the study. Furthermore, as I will discuss in Chapter 9, supplemental magnesium and calcium have been shown to lower blood pressure in individuals who have been diagnosed with hypertension.

Antioxidant deficiencies may also contribute to high blood pressure. There is increasing evidence that damage to the endothelium, or lining of the arteries, caused by reactive substances known as free radicals is an important factor in hypertension. Damage to the arteries decreases their elasticity and responsiveness to chemical signals to relax or contract. As we saw in Chapter 2, sustained contraction of the arteries and arterioles drives blood pressure up. In addition, free radical damage is a well-recognized player in atherosclerosis, which is also associated with hypertension. Antioxidant vitamins and minerals—vitamin A, beta-carotene, vitamin C, vitamin E, and selenium—negate the harmful effects of free radicals and protect the arteries. In this way antioxidants may protect against the development of hypertension.

Deficiencies in B-complex vitamins, particularly vitamin B-12, folic acid, and vitamin B-6, have also been implicated in the genesis of arterial damage and, by association, hypertension. These nutrients are important in the clearance of homocysteine, a toxic by-product of the metabolism of protein. When you have adequate amounts of these B vitamins, your body is able to break down homocysteine into harmless amino acids. If there are deficiencies in these nutrients, however—and deficiencies are quite common in our society—homocysteine builds up and damages the arteries. In recent years homocysteine has been recognized as a significant risk factor for atherosclerosis and heart disease—perhaps as important as high cholesterol. Although few studies have been conducted thus far examining the cause-effect relationship between elevated homocysteine and hypertension, there is a large and growing body of research linking elevated homocysteine levels with increased risk of atherosclerosis.

STOP SMOKING AND LIVE LONGER

Folks, the effects of smoking on your health can be summed up in one word: devastating. And if you have hypertension, the effects are doubly disastrous. More smokers die of malignant (dangerously elevated) hypertension than any other high-risk group. According to the American Heart Association, smoking is the number one cause of sudden death due to heart attack. The *New England Journal of Medicine* recently reported that hypertensive smokers are three times more likely than nonsmokers to suffer strokes and twice as likely to have heart attacks. An estimated 500,000 Americans die of smoking-related illnesses each year, and nearly a fifth of cardiovascular disease deaths are attributable to smoking. We lose another 55,000 nonsmokers yearly as a result of cardiovascular diseases due to second-hand smoke.

Although smoking may make you feel more relaxed, the nicotine in cigarettes is actually an extremely strong stimulant that constricts your arteries and reduces blood flow. And as you know, narrowed "pipes" increase pressure in the system. One study demonstrated that blood pressure increased by an average of 11 mm Hg systolic and 9 mm Hg diastolic, and heart rate increased by 43 percent, after smoking just two cigarettes!

I do understand that a smoking addiction can be terribly difficult to overcome. The addiction occurs because nicotine binds with certain neuroreceptors in the brain. As nicotine dissipates from the brain, the receptors literally cry out for more, virtually forcing you to smoke. There are, however, several prescription and nonprescription products on the market that help squelch this craving. One that has helped several of my patients stop for good is called Sulfonil. It works by binding with nicotine neuroreceptors and stifling your craving—even more effectively than the nicotine obtained from actually smoking. Sulfonil comes in capsule form and is designed to be used from the day you stop smoking to reduce nicotine cravings. You'll need to take it for only as long as your cravings persist, usually three days to two weeks. (See Appendix E for information on where to find Sulfonil.)

Once your nicotine cravings have subsided, the desire for a cigarette is no more than a habit. When you are ready to stop smoking, fill out the commitment contract (Figure 5), which I give to patients at the Whitaker Wellness Institute who have decided to quit smoking. Pledge to donate a substantial amount of money to your least favorite cause (Saddam Hussein's regime, for example) if you break your re-

Commitment Contract

I, _____ , agree to stop smoking completely for
      (your name)

_____ . If I so much as take one puff of a cigarette,
   (amount of time)

I agree to give $_____ to _____ .
   (a large sum of money)   *(your least favorite cause)*

Signed: _____ Witnessed by:_____

Date: _____

Figure 5. Smoker's Commitment Contract

solve to stop smoking. I usually recommend contracting for three
weeks, because most people feel they can commit for that amount of
time. At the end of three weeks, simply renew your commitment.

If you can't stop by yourself, find a good smoker's clinic or check
with your local chapter of the American Lung Association for help.
Whether you or a loved one has hypertension, neither of you should
be smoking. If you're serious about lowering your blood pressure, fill
out the commitment contract and follow through to achieve your goal
once and for all.

EXCESS ALCOHOL CONSUMPTION DRIVES UP BLOOD PRESSURE

Moderate, judicious use of alcohol has been demonstrated repeatedly
to have a protective effect on the heart. It raises high-density lipoprotein (HDL, the beneficial type of cholesterol), improves the viscosity,
or thickness, of the blood, and actually lowers the risk of heart attack.
But like many things in life, the benefits of alcohol hinge on balance.
Consider this major study by the Kaiser Permanente Medical Care
Program of the association between alcohol and blood pressure in
close to 84,000 of its enrollees. It was demonstrated that people having one or two drinks a day had lower blood pressure than those abstaining from alcohol altogether. More than two or three drinks per

day, however, resulted in an increase in blood pressure of an average of 10 mm Hg. Those who consumed six to eight drinks per day and also had hypertension experienced a rapid reduction in blood pressure of about 10 mm Hg when they did stop drinking.

A large-scale study on the effects of alcohol intake and cardiovascular mortality was conducted in London. The researchers assessed the benefits and risks of drinking alcohol in 6,369 patients with hypertension. They found that alcohol intake could reduce stroke and heart disease deaths—but quantity was the key once again. This study showed that the lowest mortality rate was associated with alcohol consumption of one to ten drinks per week, but more than this amount negated the health benefits of alcohol.

The consensus is that one to two drinks per day can have a protective effect on your cardiovascular system. However, I'm always a little uncomfortable espousing the health benefits of alcohol, since alcohol abuse has such widespread and devastating consequences. So please *DO NOT* take this as a recommendation to start drinking. Rather, if you like to have an occasional beer or glass of wine, enjoy it. Just remember to keep your consumption within healthy boundaries.

CHRONIC STRESS AND BLOOD PRESSURE

Chronic stress drives up blood pressure. As I explained in Chapter 2, whenever you feel threatened or stressed in any way, your adrenal glands churn out stress hormones that prepare you to fight or run like hell. Your muscles tense and your blood sugar elevates for a burst of extra energy. Your pulse and respiration rates speed up, and you become ultra alert, ready to take on whatever is threatening you. Sure, you know that you don't need to run or fight your way out of a stressful encounter with your boss or spouse, but your body is designed to react in this way regardless of the threat. Once the threat is past and the rush of stress hormones subsides, your blood pressure, pulse, and hormone levels all return to normal. But when stress piles upon stress, these hormone levels remain elevated, and your body gets stuck in that ready state. Your muscles remain tense, your pulse pounds—and your blood pressure soars. The effects of emotional stress on blood pressure have been explored in hundreds of research studies. In Chapter 14, I will give you some tips for managing the stress in your life.

In this chapter we have covered the most common causes of hypertension. In the next chapter I will tell you about other, less obvious factors that raise blood pressure.

CHAPTER 5

Less Obvious Causes of Hypertension

A 17-year-old boy was admitted to the hospital with overpowering headaches, irritability, and heavy sweating, and he was found to have severe, life-threatening hypertension (200/130 mm Hg). After a full panel of tests was taken, including urine screening and blood analysis, it was discovered that the boy was harboring dangerously high levels of mercury. Luckily, it was possible to remove this heavy metal from the boy's body, especially since it had not yet settled into his bones. Physicians immediately gave him several courses of intravenous chelation treatments, which effectively cleared out most of the mercury. His symptoms gradually subsided, and his blood pressure normalized after two months of treatment.

Obesity, dietary indiscretions, inactivity, smoking, excess alcohol, stress—these are the causes most commonly associated with hypertension. However, there are other, less evident determinants that may also increase blood pressure, even in people with none of the primary risk factors for hypertension. Many of these more subtle risk factors, including certain drugs and environmental toxins, are avoidable; it's just that few people know they are implicated in hypertension. Others, such as age, race, and sex, are beyond your control. However, it is important that you be aware of these "uncontrollable" risk factors, for if any of them apply to you, it simply means that you need to be more vigilant in following the prevention and treatment program detailed in Part II for reversing hypertension.

DRUGS THAT RAISE BLOOD PRESSURE

There are a number of drugs that cause hypertension. They're not supposed to raise blood pressure. They're prescribed for reasons completely unrelated to blood pressure—cold symptoms, for example, or pain relief. But while these drugs do indeed clear up a stuffy nose or control pain, they may also induce temporary or long-term hypertension by disrupting the body's natural blood pressure regulation systems. The good news about drug-induced hypertension is that blood pressure usually returns to normal once you stop taking the medication.

Steroids

Of all the drugs that raise blood pressure, steroids (also called corticosteroids) do so in the most dramatic way. Steroids elevate blood pressure primarily by increasing the intensity of the heartbeat. They also disturb the body's mineral balance, resulting in sodium retention and increased blood volume. These drugs should be avoided by individuals with hypertension.

Oral Contraceptives

Oral contraceptives can also cause hypertension. About 20 percent of women taking these drugs develop drug-associated hypertension. Synthetic estrogens increase blood pressure by stimulating the renin-angiotensin-aldosterone system, which, as you recall from Chapter 2, results in constriction of the arterioles and sodium and water retention. Synthetic estrogens and progesterone can also upset the body's mineral balance, resulting in increased blood volume that forces the blood pressure to rise. This is more likely to occur in older women with a predisposing condition, such as mild kidney disease or a family history of hypertension, and risk increases with duration of use. Smoking also increases the cardiovascular risks associated with oral contraceptives. Users of birth control pills have additionally been noted to have higher concentrations of copper in their blood, which is also associated with elevated blood pressure.

Nonsteroidal Anti-inflammatory Drugs

Nonsteroidal anti-inflammatory drugs, or NSAIDs, such as Motrin, Aleve, Anaprox, Advil, Naprosyn, Nalfon, and Relafen, are commonly used pain relievers that can increase blood pressure. These drugs are believed to block the synthesis of certain prostaglandins, subtle but important regulators of blood pressure. One study found that the NSAID indomethacin increased systolic blood pressure by 5 to 10 mm Hg in both normal and hypertensive subjects. A large-scale study of 94,111 Medicaid enrollees ages 65 and older also noted a relationship between elevated blood pressure and NSAIDs. Researchers compared patients who had just started taking blood pressure medications with a similar number of randomly selected enrollees not on medication and found that those who used NSAIDs were more likely to require antihypertensive drug therapy.

Many NSAIDs are now available over the counter, but if you have hypertension, you should use them with caution. If you require an occasional pain reliever for any reason, I recommend that you use aspirin or low-dose acetaminophen. But use them sparingly. Long-term use of aspirin is associated with gastrointestinal complications, including severe bleeding and even death. Acetaminophen has its own set of side effects, namely toxicity to the liver and kidneys. It should never be used in conjunction with alcohol. Consider trying a safe, natural herbal anti-inflammatory agent, such as bromelain or another enzyme, boswella, curcumin, or other herbal formulations.

Appetite Suppressants

Most nonprescription appetite suppressants or diet pills contain combinations of antihistamines and adrenergic agonists, such as ephedrine, pseudoephedrine, or caffeine. Each of these drugs directly activates the adrenal glands, stimulating the release of the fight-or-flight hormones, epinephrine and norepinephrine. As you know, these adrenal hormones increase the action and output of the heart and cause blood pressure to rise. Hypertension is one of the major side effects of these drugs, along with seizures, irregular heartbeat, agitation, and psychosis. If you have high blood pressure, you should avoid these drugs.

Nasal Decongestants and Other Cold Remedies

Decongestants lessen nasal congestion by constricting the blood vessels in the membranes of the nose and sinus. However, they also cause blood vessels to constrict throughout the body, which causes blood pressure to elevate. They should not be used by patients with hypertension for this reason. Spray decongestants are especially to be avoided, as they are easy to become dependent on, and prolonged use results in a rebound effect of increased congestion.

Narcotics

The narcotic naloxone, commonly administered to reverse anesthesia-induced respiratory depression and to treat emergency drug overdoses, can cause a substantial rise in blood pressure in hypertensive patients. Other narcotics, such as morphine, can temporarily *reduce* arterial pressure but, curiously, raise it after the brief reducing effect has worn off.

Phenylephrine

Drugs that affect the central nervous system may produce hypertension in patients of any age. For example, the topical application of phenylephrine, used in the treatment of nasal congestion sinusitis, is a significant factor in the development of hypertension among infants. Because of their immature nerve pathways, infants are much more susceptible to developing high blood pressure from this medication than are adults. This drug caused a dramatic rise in blood pressure in a 6-year-old boy we'll call Jason. During his ten-day stay in an intensive care unit, physicians became alarmed at his dramatically elevated systolic pressure, between 130 and 160 mm Hg. After they performed a panel of tests they discovered that a 10 percent phenylephrine solution was causing the problem. When the medication was withdrawn, Jason's blood pressure safely returned to normal levels.

Other Drugs That Raise Blood Pressure

Tricyclic antidepressants, monoamine oxidase inhibitors (also called MAO inhibitors), cyclosporine, and erythropoetin have all been demonstrated to elevate blood pressure. If you are taking one of these drugs—or any drug, for that matter—ask your physician about its effects on blood pressure. Also ask him or her about interactions among drugs, if you are taking more than one. Double-check with your pharmacist about the potential side effects of prescription as well as over-the-counter drugs. Drugs are too dangerous a minefield to enter without being armed with all the available information.

HIGH BLOOD PRESSURE AS A SYMPTOM OF A POISONED PLANET

For much of the past two centuries, man has treated the earth as if it were something to be conquered, consumed, bought, and sold. In the name of progress we have obliterated species and poisoned the soil, air, and water of this planet. And we're paying the price for our arrogance. High levels of toxins present in our food, air, and water supplies have brought about major unforeseen consequences, one of which is an increased incidence of hypertension. Numerous studies suggest that elevated levels of certain heavy metals in the body can significantly increase blood pressure. Lead is the most obvious offender; however, mercury, cadmium, and copper are implicated as well.

Lead

Lead is tragically harmful. This toxic metal can cause serious behavioral problems, brain damage, and learning disabilities in children who are exposed to it at an early age. And now researchers are beginning to discover a long-term repercussion of this deadly heavy metal: hypertension. In a fifty-year follow-up of thirty-five survivors of childhood lead poisoning, researcher Howard Hu uncovered an astonishingly high incidence of hypertension. Other studies have revealed that hypertension is associated with high lead concentrations in the body, especially deep within the bones.

Who gets lead poisoning, and how? We're all susceptible, since lead virtually permeates our entire environment. Even though lead-containing gasoline has been banned since 1972, our soils contain lethal amounts of this heavy metal, deposited over years of lead-laden automobile emissions. Tap water is another significant source of lead, as many older buildings have leaded or lead-soldered pipes. Another environmental source of lead is lead-based paint, banned now but still present in older buildings. According to Philip J. Landrigan, of Mount Sinai Medical Center, "Tens of millions of Americans have been exposed over the years to lead [and] adults today grew up at a time when we were still putting several thousand gallons of lead into gasoline each year." Lead blood levels are also typically elevated in chronic alcoholism, which has been linked with hypertension as well.

Lead apparently affects the renin-angiotensin-aldosterone system (RAAS) and also induces a kind of hyperactivity in the nervous system. The kidneys excrete about 90 percent of the lead absorbed in an initial exposure. However, the remaining 10 percent remains in the body, damaging the kidneys and circulating in the bloodstream, later to be stored in the bones, where it can stay for a lifetime. Ellen Silbergeld, an environment toxicologist at the University of Maryland, Baltimore, states, "The fact of the matter is that for many, many decades the environment in this country was significantly lead contaminated." Now we're paying the price.

Mercury

Mercury is a dangerous heavy metal known to weaken the immune system and damage the brain and central nervous system. Mercury also raises blood pressure, as revealed in the story of the 17-year-old boy with mercury poisoning that opened this chapter. The most significant source of mercury exposure in this country is dental fillings. Despite its widespread use in dentistry—and its unwavering support by the American Dental Association—a number of experts feel that mercury in dental amalgam fillings is anything but safe. I personally have had all my amalgam fillings removed and replaced with safer materials.

Other Heavy Metals

Copper is a trace mineral essential for collagen formation that, in the right amounts, plays a role in healthy blood pressure. Excessive copper, however, may increase systolic blood pressure. The heavy metal cadmium has also been strongly implicated in hypertension in animal studies. High serum copper and cadmium levels are common in smokers, which may be one reason smokers have higher than normal blood pressure. In fact, one study showed a group of hypertensive smokers to harbor four times the amount of toxic cadmium in their bodies than people with normal blood pressure. Another study, of 311 male workers in an alkaline battery factory, indicated a possible relationship between cadmium oxide exposure and the development of hypertension.

As researchers continue to crack the code of these heavy metal hitters, the impact of their destructive nature is beginning to be understood. Their adverse effects on blood pressure appear to be related to oxidative stress that affects the nervous system and the smooth muscle cells of the arteries. There are a number of therapies that facilitate the removal of heavy metals from the body. Chelation therapy, which the 17-year-old with mercury poisoning underwent, is one. Another is high doses of vitamin C, along with selenium and other antioxidants, which detoxify some heavy metals. Finally, it is possible to force the excretion of some metals by increasing levels of others. Zinc, for example, has been demonstrated to facilitate the removal of cadmium. (For more on chelation, see Chapter 15.)

RISK FACTORS BEYOND YOUR CONTROL

You can change your diet, begin exercising, manage stress, and avoid certain drugs and heavy metals. But unfortunately there are some risk factors over which you have no control. Some people are just more prone to hypertension than others. Age, heredity, gender, race, and poor general health can all pit the odds against us. But don't let that get you down. Remember, hypertension is primarily a lifestyle disorder. How you choose to live will ultimately determine whether or not your health is affected by these inherent risk factors.

Age

In most industrialized countries, blood pressure goes up with age. Older patients often have elevated systolic blood pressure, which has been attributed to increased peripheral resistance in the arteries. The age-related process of atherosclerosis, or hardening of the arteries (discussed in an earlier chapter), causes them to be less responsive to the natural blood-pressure-regulating hormonal and nervous system messages. There is evidence, however, that these increases in blood pressure may have more to do with other factors, such as diet, obesity, and stress, than with aging.

For example, in two populations that have been studied, the natives of New Guinea and the rural inhabitants in the Igbo-Ora area of Nigeria, hypertension is rarely present at any age—and blood pressure does not increase with age. The lifestyles of people living in these close-knit communities, however, are much different from those in the industrialized countries. These groups engage in physically demanding farming and eat traditional diets that are low in fat, protein, processed food, and sodium. Maybe it's time we stop looking at hypertension as something to be expected as we age and instead start doing something about it.

Gender

Men usually begin showing signs of hypertension in their late thirties, while women are generally unaffected until they reach the menopausal years. In fact, hypertension is about twice as common in 36-year-old men as it is in women of the same age. I suspect this has to do with a woman's estrogen and progesterone balance, which significantly protects her cardiovascular system up until menopause. More women than men actually die from hypertension, but this is attributed to their longer average life span, since blood pressure tends to rise with age.

Genetics

A family history of hypertension also increases your chances of developing this condition. If your siblings, parents, grandparents, aunts, or uncles have or had hypertension or cardiovascular problems, your likelihood of having these conditions increases. Researchers estimate that 25 to 40 percent of the variations in blood pressure among people are attributable to genetic factors, and several genes are involved. However, a genetic propensity for any condition is only that—a propensity. Whether or not the gene expresses itself and hypertension develops depends on environmental factors as well. A good example is the 235T gene variant. In people of European descent, the 235T gene is related to increased levels of angiotensinogen, which reacts with other chemicals in the blood to raise blood pressure. However, in Nigeria—where 90 percent of the people carry this gene—hypertension is extremely rare. There is obviously more at work than this single gene.

If you have a family history of hypertension, it's important that you level the playing field by doing everything in your power to avoid developing hypertension yourself. You must be extremely vigilant in following the recommendations in Part II of this book—and if you are, you'll likely be fine. Frank, a good friend of mine, has a family tree so riddled with heart disease and hypertension that not a single male on his side of the family has lived past the age of 50. I've advised Frank to adhere to this same self-care program, and at age 51 he's doing great. When the odds are against you, you must take extra steps to protect yourself.

Race

No one knows for certain why, but some ethnic groups are more prone to hypertension than others. African-Americans are the most seriously affected, developing hypertension at twice the rate of Anglo-Americans. In fact, hypertension is the number one cause of death among blacks. Death rates reveal that a full 30 percent of African-American men and 20 percent of African-American women die due to complications of high blood pressure. Other high-risk groups include Puerto Ricans, Cubans, and Mexicans. Not only are they more prone to hypertension, but its consequences are often more severe.

There has been much speculation on why this is. According to a very interesting paper entitled "The Puzzle of Hypertension in African-Americans," by Richard S. Cooper, Charles N. Rotimi, and Ryk Ward, published in *Scientific American* in 1999, one controversial but widely accepted theory has to do with that dark period in American history, the slave trade. The theory goes that because conditions were so horrendous during the trip from Africa to America on slave ships, death rates were exceptionally high. Many of the deaths were caused by salt- and water-wasting conditions, such as dehydration and diarrhea. Therefore, the tendency to retain sodium would increase survival, so more people with this genetic predisposition survived and reproduced. In modern America, this same tendency predisposes the descendants of these people to high blood pressure.

However, the authors of the paper feel this theory is too simplistic. Based on comparisons of African-Americans with Africans (who share many of the same genes but whose incidence of hypertension is extremely low), they feel that 40 to 50 percent of the increased risk of hypertension in African-Americans is likely due to a combination of lack of exercise, the unhealthy American diet, and obesity. They feel that increased sodium intake and psychological and social stressors are other important factors.

Endocrine Conditions

Hypertension is also associated with various endocrine (hormonal) problems, including Cushing's disease and thyroid disorders. Researcher Dr. Peter K. T. Pang has presented new evidence that a particular hormone called *parathyroid hypertensive factor* (PHF) plays a part in hypertension in some people. Dr. Pang first discovered that the PHF hormone was present in blood samples of hypertensive animals. When he injected a PHF antibody into hypertensive animals, their blood pressure went down. This finding is an outcome of relatively new research, but its conclusions are quite convincing. As more PHF research is done, including investigating new treatments aimed at this cause, I'm sure we will be hearing more about PHF and hypertension in the near future.

Female menopause and its male counterpart, andropause (declining testosterone levels in middle-aged men), also belong in this category, since a reduction of some sex hormones can result in increased blood pressure. High blood pressure may also develop rapidly toward the end of pregnancy, and in pregnant women who already have hypertension, it often becomes more severe. In most cases, high blood pressure that develops during pregnancy returns to normal after delivery.

Prenatal and Early Childhood Conditions

Certain prenatal and early childhood conditions may increase the tendency toward hypertension. How much a baby weighs at birth may help determine whether the child will grow up to develop high blood pressure later in life. Juno Uiterwaal and colleagues at Erasmus University in Rotterdam, the Netherlands, have found that maternal nutrition likely affects a baby's blood pressure. The lower a baby's birth weight, the higher his or her risk of developing hypertension later in life. These researchers found that infants born weighing less than 5.5 pounds are about 40 percent more likely to have high blood pressure as adults. They explained that below-normal weight may affect the development and performance of critical organs such as the heart and kidneys, which may contribute to increased risk of hypertension in adulthood.

Early nutrition is another determinant of blood pressure, as a long-term Dutch study revealed. In this clinical trial, babies fed a low-salt diet during the first six months of life grew up to have lower blood pressure in adulthood. Perhaps this has to do with the fact that without early exposure to salt they never truly acquired a taste or craving for it, and therefore used less of it later in life. In another study, 2,220 white and 1,304 African-American schoolchilden, ages 5 to 14, in Bogalusa, Louisiana, were examined for early risks of coronary heart disease. The study found that taller, obese children were more prone to higher blood pressure.

Though it certainly makes sense that childhood is where the natural history of hypertension begins, very few studies have been done on the determinants of blood pressure in the early years. Yet I am particularly concerned about the epidemic of obesity and inactivity in our children. I have always maintained that it is in our childhood that we learn how to eat, behave, and cope with daily stress. As we grow up, these patterns play themselves out to either keep us healthy or make us sick. For this reason I believe it is of vital importance that we teach our children healthy habits in these early years.

There is one more factor in the development of hypertension that I want to tell you about—insulin resistance, the topic of our next chapter. Insulin resistance is an underlying condition that increases the risk not only of hypertension but also of obesity, diabetes, and heart disease.

CHAPTER 6

Insulin Resistance: An Underlying Cause of Hypertension

George was overweight, and he carried much of that excess weight in a spare tire around his midriff. His blood sugar was in the high normal range, his cholesterol hovered around 250, his HDL cholesterol was low, and his triglycerides were over 300. He had recently been diagnosed with hypertension, and he had had several bouts of chest pain that really shook him up. George knew he was at high risk for cardiovascular disease and diabetes, and he was trying hard to make lifestyle changes to improve his health. He replaced red meat with fish and chicken and ate lots of rice, pasta, and bread. He substituted fat-free cookies, crackers, and pastries for fatty desserts and snacks. Yet despite his efforts, his weight and blood pressure remained high; his cholesterol, triglycerides, and blood sugar showed little improvement, and he felt no better.

Over the years researchers have discovered an uncanny link between hypertension and three other cardiovascular risk factors. This "deadly quartet" was given the label *syndrome X* by Stanford University Medical School professor Gerald M. Reaven, M.D., who first identified the clustering of four interrelated abnormalities: hypertension, obesity, and irregularities in blood sugar and blood lipid (cholesterol and triglycerides) levels. Syndrome X is also known as Reaven's syndrome, metabolic cardiovascular risk syndrome, and insulin resistance syndrome. No matter what you call it, these four disorders currently afflict large numbers of people in westernized societies.

Syndrome X brings with it an increased risk of heart disease and non-insulin-dependent diabetes mellitus (NIDDM; also known as type II, or maturity-onset diabetes). It is also associated with other abnormalities evident on blood tests, including high uric acid levels and two recently identified heart disease risk factors: smaller, denser LDL cholesterol and plasminogen activator inhibitor (PAI-1). Some studies even suggest an association with polycystic ovaries and breast and endometrial cancers. Who would ever have thought that hypertension could be related to so many seemingly unrelated health risks?

 CHARACTERISTICS OF SYNDROME X

- Hypertension
- Obesity, particularly in the abdominal area
- Glucose intolerance (blood sugar may be normal or slightly high while fasting but remains abnormally elevated after eating)
- Elevated triglycerides
- Increased levels of plasminogen activator inhibitor (PAI-1)
- Low HDL cholesterol and smaller, denser LDL particles
- Elevated uric acid
- Increased risk of type II diabetes mellitus
- Increased risk of atherosclerotic cardiovascular disease

It is possible—even likely—that if you have high blood pressure you have one or more of the other symptoms of syndrome X. And just as hypertension is a silent killer, syndrome X can go unnoticed for years before serious complications begin to surface. For example, my patient George, described above, presented with a classic case of syndrome X. Although he had been followed by various physicians for years, he had never been told that his many medical problems might have a common underlying connection—and a common therapy.

Syndrome X may provide a few warning signs. The most visible is abdominal obesity. Extra fat around the midriff is a common expression of syndrome X. However, you don't have to be overweight to have syndrome X. A fair number of lean individuals have this condition. Not all obese people have syndrome X. There is also a strong genetic link to this condition, so a family history of abdominal obesity, hypertension, type II diabetes, or other characteristics of syndrome X may provide clues.

It is estimated that 25 percent of Americans—including many who are apparently healthy—suffer from some degree of syndrome X. And some experts peg this number as high as 40 percent. It's important to know that if you have one manifestation of this syndrome, you may be at increased risk for others. For example, if your cholesterol and triglyceride levels are high and you have abdominal obesity, you should be screened regularly for high blood pressure, as you may be at greater risk of having hypertension than people with normal weight and blood lipids.

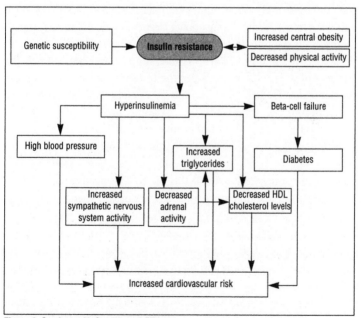

Figure 6. Syndrome X: Causes and Effects

UNDERSTANDING INSULIN RESISTANCE

The one underlying condition in all people with syndrome X—and this includes about half of those with hypertension—is insulin resistance. Insulin is your body's nutritional storage hormone, the key that opens the portals of your cells for the entry of glucose, minerals, vitamins, protein, and fat. Insulin resistance, as its name implies, is a condition in which the cells resist insulin and its attempts to usher nutrients into the cells. The body responds by producing even more insulin—sometimes 300 to 400 percent more than the average healthy person produces (a condition known as *hyperinsulinemia*).

Let's back up a bit so you can get a better picture of what insulin resistance is all about. When you eat, the process of digestion breaks carbohydrates down into small sugar molecules called glucose, which is your body's primary source of energy. Glucose is absorbed through the intestinal walls into the bloodstream, signaling the beta cells of the pancreas to secrete insulin. (A similar process takes place when you eat protein, which breaks down into amino acid and also signals an insulin response. However, glucose is key in insulin resistance, so we'll concentrate on that here.) Insulin binds to receptor sites on the surfaces of your cells and activates the transport of glucose and other nutrients into the cells. Within minutes of eating, the rate of glucose entering your cells increases fifteen to twenty times. Glucose levels in the blood then fall, and insulin production is suppressed.

Although the pancreas of an individual with insulin resistance produces adequate insulin in response to elevated blood glucose levels after eating, things fall apart at this point. The insulin receptors on the cells do not respond adequately and are unable to move sufficient amounts of glucose into the cells. Glucose remains in the bloodstream, signaling the pancreas to secrete even more insulin. This results in very high levels of both insulin and glucose. In the early stages of insulin resistance, there are no overt signs of the condition. But as it progresses and glucose metabolism remains impaired, complications arise. Type II diabetes (which is essentially severe insulin resistance) may eventually develop. Blood lipids take a turn for the worse, and free fatty acids are released from abdominal fat stores. Together, these processes endanger the cardiovascular system and increase the risk of heart disease.

HOW INSULIN RESISTANCE RAISES BLOOD PRESSURE

No one really knows exactly how insulin resistance elevates blood pressure. It may interfere with intercellular communication and thus with the body's blood-pressure-regulating systems. This could provoke and activate the sympathetic nervous system, causing the heart to pump with greater intensity and the arteries to constrict. Early research suggests involvement of the kidneys and their regulating mechanisms as well. There also appears to be a relationship between insulin resistance and several minerals involved in blood pressure control. (These four minerals and their effects on both insulin resistance and blood pressure will be covered in detail in Chapters 8 and 9.)

Regardless of the precise cause, insulin resistance is an underlying factor in approximately half of all causes of hypertension. And because of the associated components of syndrome X discussed earlier, these people are at greater risk of developing cardiovascular disease.

DIETARY ASPECTS OF INSULIN RESISTANCE

Not surprisingly, many of the dietary factors associated with hypertension also contribute to insulin resistance. Overeating of sugars and refined carbohydrates is a chief cause of this condition. In Abraham Lincoln's day, Americans consumed a modest 5 pounds of sugar a year. We now eat more than twice that much every month—about 149 pounds of sweeteners per person per year! The types of sugars we are eating may be another contributing factor to insulin resistance. The mountains of sweeteners we eat include not only white sugar (sucrose) but other sugars as well. Eighty-three of those 149 pounds are in the form of corn sweeteners, including high-fructose corn syrup, the dominant sweetener of sodas and processed foods.

And this type of fructose is known to cause insulin resistance in laboratory animals.

Refined carbohydrates are equally culpable. We are consuming unprecedented amounts of fat-free and low-fat breads, cereals, and snack foods. But these refined carbohydrates are far from healthy. They're often stripped of not only fat, but also fiber, vitamins, and virtually all nutritional value. Excessive consumption of these simple sugars and refined carbohydrates has been linked to a variety of mental and physical complaints. They are rapidly broken down into glucose and cause a much higher release of insulin than do fiber-rich, unprocessed carbohydrates, such as vegetables, legumes, fruits, and whole grains.

Eating too much fat may be another, albeit less explored, cause of insulin resistance. An excess of fatty acids circulating in the blood reduces the sensitivity of insulin receptors. Laboratory animals fed a high-fat diet will develop insulin resistance. And this is true for humans as well. Back in the 1930s Dr. H. P. Himsworth published several studies that determined that a high-fat diet could elevate blood sugar levels in normal individuals. In one of these studies, entitled "The Dietetic Factors Determining the Glucose Tolerance and Sensitivity to Insulin of Healthy Men," he found that by feeding volunteers various diets for a week before administering glucose tolerance tests, he could predictably manipulate the outcomes of those tests. The diet that raised blood sugar levels the most was extremely high in fat with restricted protein and carbohydrates—presumably by decreasing insulin sensitivity.

Inadequate consumption of vitamin- and mineral-rich plant foods is likely another dietary factor in insulin resistance. Magnesium, calcium, chromium, and vanadium have distinct roles in insulin utilization by the cells. The best food sources of these minerals are vegetables, fruits, legumes, and whole grains (along with dairy products). Due to the sad state of our diet, deficiencies in these nutrients are not uncommon. A 1995 Swiss study published in the *Journal of Hypertension* showed that hypertensive patients with insulin resistance had distinct mineral imbalances. Specifically, high levels of sodium and calcium were found in the blood, along with markedly low magnesium and potassium.

OBESITY AND INSULIN RESISTANCE

As we have discussed in previous chapters, one of the most significant risk factors for hypertension is obesity. Obesity is also a hallmark of insulin resistance. However, it's something of a chicken-and-egg relationship. While it's true that most (but not all) people with hypertension, insulin resistance, and other manifestations of syndrome X carry excess weight, it is uncertain which came first, the weight or the accompanying medical problems. The generally accepted theory is that obesity contributes to insulin resistance and its host of related conditions. However, Dr. Neil Ruderman and colleagues from Boston University Medical Center point out in a compelling 1998 paper that it is possible for an individual to be of normal weight but have the characteristics of a "metabolically obese" person—i.e., of insulin resistance. Therefore, it is conceivable that insulin resistance is the *cause* of obesity and these other conditions rather than their *effect*.

What is clear, and I touched on this earlier, is that there is a specific type of weight gain associated with insulin resistance. The best way to describe this sort of fat distribution is that the person takes on the shape of an apple—he or she carries excess fat around the midsection. This phenomenon of apple-shaped obesity has been recognized for a number of years as a risk factor for heart disease. Now there is a growing body of research linking this distribution of body fat to an increased risk of insulin resistance and diabetes as well, even in individuals who are not obese, but just a little overweight. Fat in the abdominal cells is more easily broken down than fat stored elsewhere. Free fatty acids are released into the bloodstream, where they can cause a number of problems. They increase the production of triglycerides, inhibit the action of insulin, and contribute to elevated blood sugar levels. Recent research has demonstrated that abdominal obesity coupled with an increased body mass index (BMI, or ratio of body fat to lean body mass; see Chapter 4) are associated with ill health and poorer quality of life.

▼ | ARE YOU APPLE-SHAPED?

Apple-shaped obesity can be assessed by measuring with a tape measure the narrowest point around your waist and the widest area around your hips. Divide the waist measurement by the hip measurement. If the number is greater than 0.8 in women or 0.95 in men, you have apple-shape obesity, indicating both insulin resistance and an increased risk for heart disease, hypertension, and diabetes. For example, a hip measurement of 37 inches and a waist measurement of 28 inches give a healthy ratio of 0.75, while hip and waist measurements of 36 and 37, respectively, yield an unfavorable ratio of 1.03.

An easier, though less precise way of determining this is simply to measure your waist circumference just above the tops of your hipbones. If this is more than 40 inches for men or 35 inches for women, you are at increased risk—especially if your BMI is 26 or greater. While a pear-shaped distribution of fat through the thighs and buttocks is no less unsightly, it does not increase cardiovascular risk.

OTHER CAUSES OF INSULIN RESISTANCE

Lack of exercise is a major cause of insulin resistance. Exercise dramatically increases the cells' ability to take up glucose. It actually allows the normal mechanisms of glucose transport into the cells to be bypassed to some degree, and nutrients are able to enter the muscle cells without the aid of insulin. Blood vessels in the skeletal muscles dilate during exercise, increasing delivery of nutrients to these cells. Altered level of calcium within muscle cells during exercise may also facilitate glucose entry. In addition, exercise increases levels of GLUT-4, a protein that transports glucose into skeletal muscle cells. Regular exercise keeps blood glucose levels normal and is an excellent therapy for the prevention and treatment of insulin resistance.

Genetic factors contribute to insulin resistance as well. Dr. Reaven, the "father of syndrome X," estimates that 50 percent of the tendency toward insulin resistance is genetic; the other 50 percent is lifestyle related. The Pima Indians, living near Phoenix, Arizona, are often used in studies of insulin resistance, as they are genetically predisposed to developing type II diabetes mellitus, which is a condition of severe insulin resistance. Children of parents in this population with type II diabetes often become insulin resistant by their mid-twenties, and the disorder is present in virtually all close relatives. Once the genetic basis of insulin resistance is better understood, tests may become available to help screen patients for susceptibility, allowing them to take preventive precautions early in life.

INSULIN RESISTANCE, CARDIOVASCULAR DISEASE, AND DIABETES

Because insulin resistance dramatically increases your risk of cardiovascular disease and diabetes, I want to address these two conditions briefly. Excessive circulating insulin is a clear marker for heart disease. Three major European studies have examined this relationship. In the Caerphilly, Wales, Heart Disease Study, which involved 2,512 men ages 45 to 59, a definite link between fasting plasma insulin levels and heart disease was determined—independent of all other risk factors. The Finnish Helsinki Policeman Study followed 1,059 men between the ages of 30 and 59 years for a period of five years. Researchers discovered that fatal and nonfatal heart attacks were far more common in the men with the highest insulin levels. And finally, the Paris Prospective Study, which followed 7,246 men for an average of sixty-three months, determined a direct relationship between coronary heart disease and insulin levels. This association was even more pronounced in men who were obese.

The connection between insulin resistance and diabetes is even stronger. Individuals with insulin resistance are walking a sure path toward diabetes. In fact, hypoglycemia, prediabetes, and type II diabetes are all stages of the same disease—and they all begin with insulin resistance. On average, diabetics go undiagnosed for about 7.5 years from the time insulin resistance first develops. About 14.9 million Americans have been diagnosed with type II diabetes, and another 5.4 million have it but are unaware of it. These people produce massive amounts of insulin, but it is not accepted at the insulin receptor sites. As a result, high levels of insulin and glucose circulate in the bloodstream, leading to serious health complications, such as poor circulation, blindness, kidney failure, and gangrene. Like hypertension, type II diabetes is largely the result of diet and lifestyle, and it can simply be termed *advanced, extreme,* or *end-stage insulin resistance.* In many patients, the condition is overlapped by the other disorders characteristic of syndrome X.

WHAT TO DO ABOUT INSULIN RESISTANCE

Insulin resistance and the conditions that make up the complex of syndrome X are treatable through safe, natural nutritional and lifestyle measures. Because so many of the same threads run through hypertension and insulin resistance, the treatment recommendations for lowering blood pressure will also improve insulin utilization and result in improvements in triglycerides and cholesterol. Above all, they will decrease your risk of cardiovascular disease and type II diabetes. Diet, exercise, and selected nutritional supplements are central to the treatment program I use with my patients and recommend in this book. Many of the therapies described in Part II address not only hypertension, but insulin resistance as well.

CHAPTER 7

The Dangers of Antihypertensive Drugs

John was in his thirties when he was diagnosed with hypertension and had been on three different blood pressure medications for thirty years. When he came to my clinic, he wanted to get off these drugs, or at least cut back on their doses. They made him feel listless and depressed, and although he was reluctant to discuss it, they were causing significant problems with sexual function. Worst of all, in the past ten years he had suffered three heart attacks and a stroke and had bypass surgery—all while taking drugs that were supposed to prevent these tragedies! By following the program outlined in this book, John was able to reduce his blood pressure and get off all medications. But here's the $64,000 question: Did John suffer heart attacks and a stroke because of his hypertension, or were they caused by the medications he took for thirty years?

The goal in the treatment of hypertension is to lower blood pressure in an effort to prevent the complications associated with the condition—primarily cardiovascular incidents such as heart attack, stroke, and atherosclerosis, but also memory loss and kidney damage. If this could be done with drugs that were safe, effective, and affordable, I wouldn't be writing this book. However, this is not the case. Antihypertensive medications are expensive (Americans spend an estimated $10 billion a year on drugs to lower blood pressure), have numerous side effects (some of them life-threatening, as I will describe in this chapter), and don't always work (only 27 percent of patients with hypertension have their blood pressure under control—

though this figure includes everyone with hypertension, regardless of whether or not they are taking drugs).

This doesn't mean such drugs don't have their merits. There is a general consensus that the incidence of stroke has been reduced by the use of antihypertensive drugs. A short course of drugs, used temporarily to bring down severely elevated blood pressure, is sometimes necessary. Furthermore, in some patients—even some of my patients—blood pressure remains elevated in spite of strict adherence to the measures outlined in this book. For these patients, longer-term use of blood-pressure-lowering drugs is appropriate.

My beef with the approach conventional medicine takes toward hypertension, however, is the idea that drugs are seen as the one and only ticket to normal blood pressure. If you have been diagnosed with hypertension, chances are you are taking, or have been prescribed, a drug to lower your blood pressure. Prescribing drugs is what doctors do. It's at the heart of medical education, and the pharmaceutical industry is the engine that drives conventional medicine. Because of their enthusiasm for drugs, physicians often neglect to counsel patients about alternative therapies for lowering blood pressure. This simply flies in the face of current research.

The latest recommendations of the Joint National Committee on the Prevention, Detection, Evaluation, and Treatment of High Blood Pressure (JNC VI) include a three- to six-month trial of nondrug therapies before beginning medications for patients with mild (stage 1, 140–159 systolic, 90–99 diastolic) to moderate (stage 2, 160–179 systolic and 100–109 diastolic) hypertension. Furthermore, seven large, well-respected studies have demonstrated that antihypertensive drugs offer no significant protection against heart disease in patients with mild to moderate hypertension. Beginning a lifelong course of drugs without thoroughly exhausting safer, saner measures is, in my opinion, unconscionable.

In this chapter I will cover the major categories of antihypertensive drugs. We will discuss how these drugs work—information you'll probably get from your doctor—as well as potential side effects and adverse reactions of which you may not be aware. It is not my intention to frighten you or make you nervous about the drugs you may be taking. Under no circumstances should you discontinue any drug without the consent and supervision of your physician. However, I believe that the bias toward drugs often blinds us to their shortcomings. I merely want to present you with the big picture.

ALL DRUGS HAVE SIDE EFFECTS

Blood-pressure-lowering drugs are big business. An estimated 20 million Americans take medications to lower their blood pressure, and they spend approximately $10 billion per year on these drugs. No other industry produces substances as expensive and, at the same time, as dangerous as the pharmaceutical business—not even the firearms industry. Of the 8,000,000 people admitted to hospitals each year, 2,240,000 of them are brought in for adverse drug reactions.

These patients are not sick from illicit drug use or overdoses of medication. They are suffering from the negative side effects of drugs prescribed by their doctors—drugs they were using exactly as their doctors recommended. This is known as *iatrogenic illness.* (*Iatrogenic* comes from the ancient Greek word *iatros*, which translates into "doctor," while *genic* means "producing" or "caused by.") Iatrogenic illnesses are ailments that stem from medical treatment. Adverse drug reactions account for most iatrogenic illnesses, and they can range from mild symptoms such as headaches or drowsiness to serious organ damage and death. The adverse effects of prescription drugs are responsible for over 100,000 deaths a year—more than twice as many as the 45,000 deaths that result each year from motor vehicle accidents.

A 1998 study published in the *Journal of the American Medical Association* showed that adverse drug reactions to prescription drugs used as prescribed are the fourth to sixth leading cause of death in this country (depending on the statistical database used), after heart disease, cancer, stroke, and possibly before chronic obstructive pulmonary disease and accidents. The true figure is likely even higher since many of the deaths attributed to heart disease and other ailments are actually caused by prescription medications.

While these statistics seem unbelievable at first glance, they become more credible when you take a cold, hard look at the unique characteristics of drugs. Drugs are *xenobiotic* agents (*xenos* means "stranger"), substances not found in nature. Because no one can patent something that Mother Nature has already created, pharmaceutical companies spend millions of dollars creating and marketing alien substances that they *can* patent. These xenobiotics alter biological systems in an attempt to bring about a desired effect—but do so only by causing side effects that are sometimes more troublesome and dangerous than the ailment for which they were prescribed.

The annals of medicine are filled with references to drugs that have fallen to the wayside because they turned out to have unacceptably dangerous side effects. These medications may well have done what they were intended to do, but in the process they so adversely affected other systems in the body that they caused serious injury and even death. The treatment was more deadly than the cure. I am not suggesting that we turn back the clock and throw out all medications. As a traditionally trained M.D., I am well aware of the lifesaving benefits of a number of drugs, and I use some of them in my medical practice. But even the best of drugs by their very nature will have unwanted side effects. The bottom line is that drugs are sometimes necessary, but there is no question that they are seriously overused. Whenever there is an alternative therapy, such as the program described in this book, for reversing hypertension, my advice is to jump on it, regardless of the efforts that may be involved.

ANTIHYPERTENSIVE DRUGS AND THEIR SIDE EFFECTS

The antihypertensive drugs we will discuss in this chapter have all been proven effective at lowering blood pressure. No one class of drugs works for all patients—all appear to work in 50 to 60 percent of the patients who try them. I hope I've made it clear that there is no one underlying cause of hypertension. Many factors are at work, and each type of drug addresses specific blood-pressure-regulating mechanisms.

All drugs have side effects, although some people tolerate them better than others. Some, for example, may interfere with sexual function, while others may contribute to depression or cause a dry cough. And although these drugs do lower blood pressure, several well-designed clinical trials have shown that antihypertensive drugs may not protect against heart disease—the very reason they're prescribed in the first place. In fact, some have been linked to an increased risk of death!

Let's take a close look at these drugs and I'll explain how they reduce blood pressure and what undesirable effects they can have on your health.

DIURETICS CAUSE NUTRIENT LOSSES

Diuretics, also called water pills, have been used as a treatment for hypertension for almost fifty years. Considered to be the standard first-line drug therapy for hypertension, diuretics stimulate the kidneys to excrete more salt and fluid. This reduces blood pressure by decreasing blood volume and thus pressure against the "pipes." Unfortunately, while excess sodium and water are flushed out of the body, a host of essential water-soluble nutrients are lost at the same time.

Long-term use of diuretics increases the possibility of severe life-threatening heart arrhythmias and raises levels of cholesterol, triglycerides, and other lipids in the blood. Studies have demonstrated that patients taking diuretics may have an increased risk of death due to heart attack or sudden death due to loss of important minerals involved in regulating the electrical activity of the heart. Other potential side effects include kidney damage, fatigue, muscle cramping, faintness, and increased incidence of gallstones. Diabetics with hypertension should discuss alternatives to diuretics with their doctors. These drugs may further reduce the diabetic's already suboptimal mineral reserves, leading to increased risk of diabetic complications of the nerves and blood vessels. Long-term use of diuretics can also cause elevations in blood uric acid levels, which can lead to gout, as they did in a 74-year-old patient we'll call Nancy.

Nancy was hospitalized after complaining of a one- to two-week history of pain, swelling, and redness in three of her fingers. Her physician suspected an infection; however, all of Nancy's tests came up negative. Three months prior to the onset of her symptoms, Nancy had started taking the diuretic furosemide for edema, or fluid retention. Her dosage was gradually increased to 320 milligrams per day, but on that dose she reported feeling "washed out." She was eventually admitted to the hospital, where she was found to have severe dehydration and low blood pressure. Blood tests showed Nancy's level of uric acid and creatinine to be abnormally high, indicative of compromised kidney function and gout. With more testing, physicians found that her joints contained large numbers of the needle-shaped crystals typical of gout. When the diuretic was stopped, her edema, which had cleared up, did not recur. Nancy's blood tests rapidly returned to normal, and within four weeks all symptoms of gout had disappeared completely.

The most commonly prescribed drugs of this class are thiazide diuretics. They are, in my opinion, the most dangerous of the diuretics. Extensive research has uncovered the dangers of these drugs. The Multiple Risk Factor Intervention Trial (MRFIT) was a double-blind, placebo-controlled study carried out in the late 1970s and early 1980s, involving over 12,800 men considered to be at high risk for heart attack because of high blood pressure, elevated serum cholesterol, and smoking. The purpose of the study was to compare the effects of aggressive drug treatment (mainly thiazide diuretics) on these patients with the effects of minimal drug treatment. The results sent shock waves through the medical community. MRFIT found that stepped-up drug treatment *did* lower blood pressure, but there was no evidence of decreased death rate. Even more disturbing: Aggressive drug therapy for men with mild hypertension (those with a diastolic of 90 to 94) resulted in an *increase* in death rate. Only those study participants with diastolic readings above 100 showed a decreased rate of death with aggressive intervention.

Another study of thiazide diuretics, conducted by the British Medical Research Council and published in 1985, found that 33 percent of the patients taking these drugs had irregular heartbeats during the day and 20 percent had them at night. In comparison, 20 percent of the placebo group had irregular heartbeats during the day, and only 9 percent had them at night. The study directly linked this increase in irregular heartbeats to low serum potassium, which occurs in 10 to 50 percent of patients taking thiazide diuretics.

In an attempt to correct the potassium problem, pharmaceutical companies developed a new breed of potassium-sparing diuretics. These drugs block the action of aldosterone, a hormone that causes the kidneys to reabsorb more sodium. (See the description of the renin-angiotensin-aldosterone system in Chapter 2.) At the same time, aldosterone increases the excretion of potassium, so blocking its action does one thing that the thiazide diuretics do not do—it helps the body retain potassium. Potassium-sparing diuretics sometimes do too good a job and result in elevated potassium levels. This can cause heart arrhythmias and other problems, particularly in patients with kidney disease. In addition, because they are weaker, potassium-sparing diuretics are often used in combination with other diuretics.

Potassium-sparing diuretics do not, however, address the loss of other water-soluble nutrients lost in the excessive urination caused by the drugs themselves. One of the most significant nutrient losses caused by potassium-sparing diuretics is magnesium. Magnesium is critical for the regulation of normal blood pressure and for overall healthy heart function, as we will discuss in Chapter 9. One study, published in the *British Medical Journal*, linked magnesium losses caused by long-term diuretic therapy to an increase in heart failure.

Loop diuretics, the final class of diuretics, are also the strongest. Loop diuretics remove more sodium from the kidneys than other diuretics, and they are often used when thiazides don't do the job. They are commonly prescribed for patients with heart failure or kidney failure, for whom fluid retention is a life-threatening condition. Because they are so strong, loop diuretics can lead to dehydration, which further interferes with blood pressure control.

Dr. Norman Kaplan, a noted authority on hypertension and head of the Hypertension Division at the University of Texas Southwestern Medical School, warned in an interview with the *Medical Tribune*, "My major recommendation to physicians [prescribing diuretics for hypertension] is to watch the potassium and the cholesterol levels. Present evidence suggests that even a mild degree of hypokalemia [low serum potassium] poses a potential hazard, which may become real when people are under stress. We are seeing many more sudden deaths in patients who have been on diuretics and are hypokalemic [potassium deficient]." I consider diuretics to be overprescribed, and I highly discourage their long-term use. Salt restriction and/or increased intake of potassium work equally well in many patients, and the best diuretic in the world, believe it or not, is water. (See Chapters 8 and 12.)

BETA-BLOCKERS WEAKEN THE HEART

Beta-blockers, among the most widely prescribed medications for hypertension, act on two fronts to lower blood pressure. First, they reduce the heart's pumping intensity by binding to certain receptors in the heart muscle cells called *beta adrenergic receptors*. This blocks the ability of the heart to respond to epinephrine (also called adrenaline), an adrenal hormone released in response to stress, which causes the heart to beat faster and with more force. Second, beta-blockers inhibit the kidney's release of renin, an enzyme that sets the RAAS pathway into motion. (See pages 24–25 for a discussion of RAAS.) These drugs therefore prevent RAAS-induced constriction of the blood vessels and retention of sodium and water in the blood, keeping blood pressure in the normal range. Because beta-blockers have a broad range of effects on the cardiovascular system, they are also used for other cardiovascular conditions, including angina (chest pain) and arrhythmia (irregular heartbeat).

The versatility of beta-blockers is not without cost. Beta-blockers have more potential side effects than any other medication for hypertension, including impaired circulation, cold extremities, palpitations, fatigue, insomnia, dizziness, and nausea. Beta-blockers can also cause sexual dysfunction and contribute to depression. Some beta-blockers may also cause constriction of the airways and should not be used by patients with asthma. Patients with diabetes, liver or kidney disease, or other cardiovascular disorders such as congestive heart failure (CHF) should discuss with their doctors the contraindications for the use of beta-blockers. In addition, beta-blockers are not very well tolerated by older patients. According to a 1998 review of ten clinical trials involving 16,000 elderly patients, published in the *Jour-*

nal of the American Medical Association, these drugs control blood pressure in only one-third of elderly patients who try them. Almost two-thirds of such patients discontinue beta-blockers due to adverse side effects.

Furthermore, because these drugs decrease cardiac output, they limit your ability to exercise—a definite negative for patients with hypertension. Because long-term use of beta-blockers weakens the heart muscle, prolonged use is decidedly dangerous. After several years of use, the heart muscle may significantly weaken, and in the long run, these drugs may increase the risk of heart failure. I strongly suspect that beta-blockers are one of the causes of our nation's increase in CHF. According to American Heart Association statistics, 377,000 people were hospitalized for CHF in 1979, a number that by 1996 had grown to 870,000—an increase of over 130 percent! Thirty years ago, patients with congestive heart failure invariably had a history of heart attacks that destroyed sections of their heart muscle and rendered it incapable of pumping blood. Yet today patients with no prior history of heart attacks are developing congestive heart failure. In my opinion, the obvious reason for this increase is the overuse of beta-blockers.

Here's what the *Physicians' Desk Reference* (PDR), which is the doctor's prescription drug bible, has to say about one representative beta-blocker, Lopressor:

WARNINGS

Cardiac Failure: Sympathetic stimulation is a vital component supporting circulatory function in congestive heart failure, and beta-blockade carries the potential hazard of further depressing myocardial contractility and precipitating more severe failure.

In Patients Without a History of Cardiac Failure: Continued depression of the myocardium with beta-blocking agents over a period of time can, in some cases, lead to cardiac failure.

ADVERSE REACTIONS

Cardiovascular: Shortness of breath and bradycardia [heart rate below 60] have occurred in approximately 3 of 100 patients. Cold extremities; arterial insufficiency, usually of the Raynaud type; palpitations; congestive heart failure; peripheral edema; and hypotension have been reported in about 1 of 100 patients.

An important note: Cessation of beta-blockers must be done gradually and under the supervision of a physician. If these drugs are stopped abruptly, a dangerous rebound effect could occur that could precipitate a heart attack.

▼ DIURETICS AND BETA-BLOCKERS MAY INCREASE RISK OF SUDDEN DEATH

According to a 1995 study published in the *Annals of Internal Medicine,* non-potassium-sparing diuretics and beta-blockers may increase the risk of sudden cardiac death. Researchers from Erasmus University Medical Center in Rotterdam, the Netherlands, examined the medical records of 257 patients who had died suddenly while taking drugs for high blood pressure and compared them with those of 257 living patients also taking antihypertensive drugs. They discovered that patients taking thiazide or loop diuretics had double the risk of sudden death compared with those taking potassium-sparing diuretics. The research team also found that patients taking beta-blockers were 1.7 times as likely to succumb to sudden cardiac death as patients taking other blood-pressure-lowering medications. They concluded that this increased risk of death may offset the benefits of these drugs.

ACE INHIBITORS BLOCK THE FORMATION OF ANGIOTENSIN

Angiotensin-converting enzyme (ACE) inhibitors reduce blood pressure by blocking the conversion of angiotensin I to angiotensin II. You may recall that although angiotensin I has no adverse effects, it reacts with ACE to produce angiotensin II, which causes the blood vessels to constrict and raises blood pressure. When the action of ACE is blocked, less angiotensin II is produced, the arteries relax and dilate slightly, and blood flows more freely with less pressure through the circulatory system. This also results in suppression of the production of aldosterone, so more sodium and fluid are excreted by the kidneys. ACE inhibitors are particularly effective for patients with high levels of renin, the enzyme released by the kidneys that combines with angiotensinogen to produce angiotensin I. Renin can be measured by a blood test, which may be helpful in determining who may benefit most from these drugs.

ACE inhibitors are becoming more popular for the treatment of hypertension. Their most dangerous—though quite rare—side effect is an acute swelling of the face, tongue, lips, vocal cords, and extremities. This condition can be life threatening, and medical help should be sought immediately if it occurs. Other potential side effects include altered sense of taste, indigestion, and alterations in levels of trace minerals in the blood. Anyone with lung or kidney disease should avoid these drugs. They may also cause birth defects, so they must be strictly avoided by women who are pregnant or likely to become pregnant.

In addition, up to 20 percent of all people who take ACE inhibitors develop a persistent dry cough. One patient, Marsha, developed a dry, irritating cough after she began taking Capoten. When she stopped taking the drug, her cough spontaneously disappeared. When doctors readministered the drug, it recurred. This "test" was performed twice, and each time Marsha stopped taking the medication her cough disappeared. The reason for this side effect? ACE inhibitors can raise the blood levels of *bradykinin*, a naturally occurring protein that causes contractions of smooth muscle. Bradykinin can also trigger bronchoconstriction and asthmatic symptoms in some patients, which explains why Marsha's cough persisted with the medication.

CALCIUM CHANNEL BLOCKERS RELAX
THE BLOOD VESSELS

The smooth muscle cells of our arteries contain minuscule channels called *calcium channels*. When calcium flows into these channels the muscles contract and cause the arteries to narrow, thus driving up blood pressure. Calcium channel blockers lower blood pressure by filling these channels and preventing excess calcium from entering the cells. This relaxes the artery walls and allows them to dilate, thereby reducing blood pressure. In addition, some calcium channel blockers slow the heart rate somewhat, which also contributes to lower blood pressure.

There are two types of calcium channel blockers. The short-acting drugs work quickly, usually within thirty minutes, but their effects are transient, so they must be taken several times a day. Long-acting calcium channel blockers are slower to work, but their effects are sustained for a longer duration. This makes them superior to short-acting drugs for lowering blood pressure.

Like all drugs, calcium channel blockers are designed to alter some system in your body to produce a desired effect. And when you interfere with a natural system you can expect trouble. As Susan Ross pointed out in the *Clinical Pharmacy Review* in 1995, "Calcium is an essential component in a variety of cardiovascular functions. The contractile processes of the heart and smooth muscle, initiation of action potentials in cardiac conducting cells, and the storage and use of energy in the myocardium are all dependent on the presence of calcium." Yes, calcium channel blockers accomplish their desired effect, but they do so only by blocking essential functions of the heart and blood vessel cells. They therefore invite a long list of life-threatening side effects.

Possible side effects caused by calcium channel blockers include potassium loss, elevated serum cholesterol, rash, headaches, dizziness, nausea, swelling in the lower extremities, low blood pressure, and constipation. Calcium channel blockers also appear to adversely affect the heart muscle itself. In addition, they interfere with normal carbohydrate metabolism, which is why I strongly discourage diabetics from using these drugs.

Researcher Bruce Psaty, M.D., was among the first to expose some of the more serious side effects of these drugs. In a double-blind study sponsored by the National Institutes of Health, Dr. Psaty compared 623 hypertensive patients having a history of heart attack with a control group of 2,032 hypertensive patients who had not suffered a heart attack. He found that individuals on calcium channel blockers experienced a 60 percent increase in myocardial infarction when compared with subjects on diuretics or beta-blockers. While commenting that the drugs posed little risk over the short term, Dr. Psaty stated, "From the point of view of public health in the United States, the long-term safety and efficacy of these drugs is an important question." When he presented his findings at the American Heart Association's annual epidemiology meeting, he explained the statistics this way: In the course of a year, heart attacks might strike about 10 of every 1,000 people being treated for hypertension with other drugs. This risk might rise to 16 of every 1,000 people being treated with calcium channel blockers—a 60 percent increase!

There is a possibility that calcium channel blockers may have cancer-causing effects as well, most likely by altering apoptosis, an important cellular mechanism for destroying abnormal cells. Researchers at the Catholic University in Rome evaluated 5,052 hypertensive patients ages 71 years or older who lived in Massachusetts, Iowa, or Connecticut. When they compared those taking calcium channel blockers with other participants, they found that older hypertensive patients taking calcium channel blockers developed cancer at about twice the rate of similar patients taking the other blood-pressure-lowering drugs. In this study, which was published in *The Lancet* in 1996, the most common cancers associated with calcium channel blockers included lung, urinary tract, colorectal, prostate, and breast cancers. Although more recent studies have shown no relationship between these drugs and cancer risk, I recommend that patients minimize their use of these potentially harmful drugs.

▼ | GRAPEFRUIT JUICE AND SOME DRUGS DON'T MIX

Think again before you belt down your medications with grapefruit juice. Naringenin, a flavonoid in grapefruit juice, increases the absorption and slows the metabolism of certain drugs, including the calcium channel blockers verapamil, nifedipine, and felodipine. This natural plant compound, which interferes with the liver's ability to detoxify and eliminate these drugs, intensifies their effects and causes them to remain in your system for prolonged periods. You should never take these calcium channel blockers with grapefruit juice, and it should be avoided for at least two hours before and two hours after taking these medications. Orange juice and other citrus juices do not affect these medications. Discuss possible food-drug interactions with your doctor.

OTHER DRUGS FOR HYPERTENSION

There are a few other classes of drugs used in the treatment of hypertension. *Alpha-blockers*, in a manner similar to beta-blockers, interfere with signals sent via the sympathetic nervous system to speed up and intensify the heartbeat. However, they act on alpha receptors, which are found in the blood vessels as well as the heart. By blocking alpha receptors, they interfere with the activity of norepinephrine, causing the heart to beat with less force and the blood vessels to relax, resulting in a lowering of blood pressure.

Because alpha-blockers inhibit natural blood pressure regulation mechanisms, they may cause dizziness and light-headedness when the person taking them rises from a reclining or sitting position. Other side effects include headache, weakness, nausea, and erectile dysfunction. Because they also relax muscles in the urinary tract, they are sometimes prescribed for men with benign prostatic hyperplasia, or noncancerous swelling of the prostate that results in impaired urine flow.

Central adrenergic inhibitors are also occasionally prescribed for hypertension, although only in specific circumstances. These drugs lower blood pressure by acting on the central nervous system to block signals from the brain that instruct the arteries to narrow and the heart rate to speed up. Potential side effects of these drugs include erectile dysfunction, cognitive dysfunction, headaches, weight gain, depression, and other psychological disorders. They may also have a sedative effect and can cause serious fatigue and drowsiness.

A new class of antihypertensive drugs that has emerged in the last few years is *angiotensin II receptor blockers*. These drugs also work on the RAAS, the same system that ACE inhibitors dampen, but, as their name implies, they directly address angiotensin II. Side effects and contraindications are similar to those of ACE inhibitors with one exception. These drugs do not increase levels of bradykinin, the substance responsible for the dry cough that so many patients on ACE inhibitors experience.

▼ BLOOD PRESSURE DRUGS CAN WORSEN EYE DISEASE

Doctors who advise patients to take their antihypertensive medicine at bedtime may be doing them a great disservice, according to researcher Sohan Singh Hayreh. Taking blood pressure medication at night can worsen some eye diseases, causing sudden or partial vision loss or promoting gradual blindness. Glaucoma, the nation's second leading cause of blindness, afflicts 1.5 million to 3 million Americans, and 40,000 to 120,000 have been blinded by this condition. Characterized by high fluid pressure in the eyes, glaucoma gradually damages the optic nerve and results in blindness if untreated. According to Dr. Hayreh, the sharp drop in blood pressure that occurs after taking antihypertensive drugs at night can aggravate glaucoma.

It can also trigger optic nerve stroke, sudden damage to the optic nerve caused by a rapid drop in blood pressure, which deprives the optic nerve of vital blood and oxygen. This, in turn, causes abrupt injury to the eye or aggravates existing damage. Patients wake up with partial or total vision loss that may be temporary or permanent. In a study of 150 patients with a history of either optic nerve stroke or glaucoma, Dr. Hayreh found these patients had a 26 to 34 percent drop in blood pressure during sleep, compared with the 7 to 18 percent drop that most people experience.

If you are currently taking antihypertensive medication and your doctor has advised you to take it before bedtime, I strongly recommend you talk to your physician about changing your medication schedule.

IN SUMMARY

As the scientific data in this chapter makes perfectly clear, antihypertensive drugs can have a host of unpleasant and potentially lethal side effects. For many patients with mild to moderate hypertension—and this includes 80 percent of all patients—blood pressure can be controlled by nondrug means. Many of the people who come to my clinic are taking one or more medications to control their blood pressure, and most have been told they would be taking these drugs for the rest of their lives. This need not be the case, and I'm out to prove it. Most drug-dependent patients can gradually taper off their medications under the supervision of their doctor, while at the same time starting on a healthy diet, regular exercise, nutritional supplementation, and a stress-reduction regimen to correct the underlying causes of their elevated blood pressure.

My goal is to help you get your blood pressure down safely without the use of drugs. In my medical practice, I resort to medication only when absolutely necessary. For example, if I am dealing with a patient whose blood pressure is dangerously high, I might resort to drug therapy to bring the pressure down. But even in these cases I try to prescribe only one medication and wean the patient off the drug just as quickly as possible. Since I began my practice over twenty-five years ago, I've been looking for a better, safer means of managing hypertension. And as thousands of my patients can attest—and as you will read in Part II of this book—I have found it.

Important Note: After reading this chapter, you may be inclined to immediately stop your antihypertensive medications. Please *do not* do this! If you are on a drug treatment program for hypertension, you need to work very closely with your physician to gradually reduce your dosages as you progress with the natural therapies that I recommend in this book.

PART II

SAFE, EFFECTIVE NATURAL THERAPIES FOR HYPERTENSION

Welcome to the most exciting part of this book! The natural therapies we will be discussing in the remainder of this book are scientifically proven and clinically tested, and have been successfully used with thousands of patients at the Whitaker Wellness Institute. Nonpharmacological approaches to the management of hypertension are now being recommended in even the most conservative medical journals. Even the Joint National Committee on the Prevention, Detection, Evaluation, and Treatment of High Blood Pressure (JNC), a guiding body of physicians and researchers who specialize in hypertension, has seen the light. In their sixth and most recent report (JNC VI, issued in 1997), they recommended lifestyle modifications as the primary treatment for most patients with high normal blood pressure (130–139/85–89). They also suggested a twelve-month trial of lifestyle changes for patients with stage 1 hypertension (140–159/90–99) before drug therapy is implemented.

JNC VI LIFESTYLE MODIFICATION GUIDELINES FOR THE TREATMENT OF HIGH BLOOD PRESSURE

- Weight loss
- Limited alcohol intake (1 ounce of ethanol per day, which equates to 24 ounces of beer, 10 ounces of wine, or 2

ounces of 100-proof hard liquor—or half this amount for
women and people of lower weight)
- Aerobic exercise (30 to 45 minutes most days of the week)
- Reduced sodium intake (less than 2,400 milligrams sodium
  or 6,000 milligrams sodium chloride)
- Increased dietary potassium intake (about 3,400 milli-
  grams per day)
- Adequate dietary calcium and magnesium intake
- Smoking cessation
- Reduced intake of saturated fat and cholesterol

Many doctors underestimate the power of these lifestyle changes
and their patients' motivation and ability to implement them. They
don't spend enough time educating their patients about how to incorporate these measures into their daily lives—hardly surprising in
this age of ten-minute HMO visits. As a result, patients make meager
efforts and show little improvement. So doctors often plunge right
into prescribing medications. Furthermore, because the JNC VI
guidelines mention dietary changes but include no recommendations
for nutritional supplements, patients continue to receive inadequate
intakes of certain important nutrients. As a result, improvements are
slower and less dramatic than they would be on a more comprehensive program that guarantees adequate nutrition.

Let's get down to the business of reversing hypertension. In the remainder of this book I will describe for you in detail the therapies I
have been recommending to my patients with high blood pressure for
the past twenty-five years. They may sound simple, even simplistic—
taking nutritional supplements, making changes in your diet, drinking
a lot of water, exercising regularly, and managing stress. But as you
will see, the effectiveness of these natural therapies is backed by an
impressive body of scientific literature.

I've done everything I can think of to make this program easy to
implement and easy to stick to. I've streamlined my supplement recommendations. I've worked with the chef and the nutritionist at the
Whitaker Wellness Institute to create easy-to-prepare, delicious
recipes so you won't feel hungry or deprived—nor be required to
spend hours in the kitchen. I've consulted with our exercise physiol-

ogist to design an exercise program that most people should be able to follow. The only unknown in the equation is you. Motivation and consistency are the cards that you bring to the table. I do know, however, that your proactive stance in seeking out more information on your condition substantially increases your likelihood of being able to turn your lifestyle around and reverse hypertension.

Let's get started, and remember, thousands have traveled the path you're starting on, and their lives have improved dramatically as a result.

CHAPTER 8

Salt and Potassium: Dynamic Duo for Healthy Blood Pressure

Bob is an engineer with a twenty-five-year history of hypertension. Over the years he had also been on a number of antihypertensive medications, jumping from one to another as side effects became intolerable. An avid reader and researcher, he had also tried over a dozen nondrug approaches to lowering blood pressure without success. In 1998, in desperation and determination, he decided to revisit one of these alternative approaches. He made a concerted effort to dramatically increase his potassium intake. He did this by eating more fruits and vegetables and supplementing with small doses of potassium gluconate. At the same time he began a gradual tapering of his medications, while carefully monitoring his blood pressure several times a day. He immediately noticed a downward trend in his blood pressure, and after three weeks, he was able to get off his medications altogether while his blood pressure remained in the 120–130/80–90 range.

Although Bob no longer takes potassium supplements, he has kept up his potassium intake by eating lots of plant foods. Today, almost two years later, Bob's blood pressure remains in the normal range, averaging what he describes as a "boring" 110/70—without medications.

Chinese emperor Su Wen observed in 2600 B.C. that "If too much salt is used in food the pulse hardens. . . . The corresponding illness makes the tongue curl up and the patient unable to speak." Thus, it has been recognized for more than 4,500 years that excess salt in the diet causes hypertension ("the pulse hardens") and stroke ("the patient unable to speak"). And for years physicians have been telling their hypertensive patients to cut down on salt, or to cut it out of their diets completely. However, this prescription is now being challenged, as new avenues of research are recognizing the importance of sodium in various physiological functions. The purpose of this chapter is to tell you the other half of the story. Elevations in blood pressure are caused by *imbalances* in sodium and other minerals, not by excess sodium alone. So let's begin by taking a look at the important role sodium plays in your health.

Literally every cell in your body requires sodium to function properly. Sodium governs a number of important physiological processes. It controls the volume of extracellular fluid (fluid outside the cells), helps pump glucose through the intestinal walls and into the bloodstream, and aids digestion by assisting in the production of hydrochloric acid. Sodium also regulates the body's water balance and blood volume. Perhaps most important, sodium is an important part of the energy system in each of your cells—it gives cells the electrical charge they need for optimal function.

A TALE OF TWO MINERALS

Every cell in your body has its own electrical system, which is powered by sodium. Sodium is an essential electrolyte, a substance that carries an electric charge and conducts electricity when dissolved in water. It is required for two major energy-producing and -storing processes that occur in your cells: the *sodium-potassium pump* and the *sodium battery*.

The sodium ion carries a positive electric charge. It is naturally more concentrated on the outside of your body's cells, in the blood and body fluids. Here it coexists in a special relationship with other positively charged minerals, including potassium, magnesium, and calcium. Because opposites—positive and negative charges—attract, sodium is motivated to move from the outside of a cell to the inside, which is

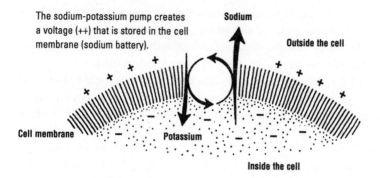

Figure 7. The Sodium-Potassium Pump and the Sodium Battery

negatively charged. While trying to get into the cells, sodium partici-
pates in an electrochemical exchange process with another charged
ion, potassium. Both sodium and potassium are positively charged, so
they are in constant competition to get inside the negatively charged
cell. Ideally, potassium has the upper hand (95 percent of the body's
potassium resides inside the cells) while sodium steps aside, moving to
the outside of the cell in exchange for the incoming potassium.

This shifting of sodium and potassium is a sort of "ionic dance"
across the cell membranes that creates an electrical potential. This is
the *sodium-potassium pump,* and the electricity produced by this action is the driving force of your muscles, organs, and many other bodily functions. The sodium-potassium pump creates a voltage, a true
electrical charge, along the cell membrane. The stored electrical potential of the positively charged sodium ions that collect on the membrane of the cells is called the *sodium battery.*

The sodium battery runs other cellular processes. One that is particularly important in hypertension is the *calcium pump,* which maintains the proper ratio of calcium inside and outside the cells. As we
saw in our discussion of calcium channel blocker drugs in Chapter 7,
an excess of intracellular calcium in the smooth muscle cells of the arteries causes them to contract and blood pressure to rise. When the
sodium battery is charged up, it keeps the calcium pump running so
the cell membranes keep out excess calcium and blood pressure re-

mains normal. In addition to raising blood pressure, elevated calcium levels inside the cells also interfere with their ability to let glucose enter in the presence of insulin—in other words, they contribute to insulin resistance.

Unfortunately, these important cellular processes can be disturbed by an imbalance of sodium and potassium in your system (as well as of calcium and magnesium, which we will discuss in the next chapter). What causes such imbalances? Too much dietary salt and too little dietary potassium, a state not unusual in people who consume the typical American diet, which is high in sodium from processed foods and low in potassium from fruits and vegetables. Years of dietary indiscretions eventually prevent the kidneys from properly clearing excess sodium. As potassium loses the upper hand, sodium builds up in the system, disrupting the sodium-potassium pump. The sodium battery—just like the battery in your car—doesn't get charged up properly and eventually runs down. As a result, cellular processes go awry. Furthermore, excess sodium, which causes the body to hold on to water, brings the blood volume up. The end result is extra fluid pressing against the pipes—high blood pressure. To reverse the situation, we must increase our potassium intake and cut back on sodium.

THE POWER OF POTASSIUM

Potassium may be the single most important nutrient for controlling sodium levels and normalizing blood pressure. It lowers blood pressure by balancing the sodium-potassium ratio and keeping the sodium battery primed, which keeps the smooth muscles of the arteries relaxed. This mineral also helps normalize the blood-pressure-regulating hormones in the kidneys and naturally promotes the excretion of excess sodium. In addition, potassium helps maintain a regular heartbeat and proper fluid balance in the cells, and it assists in the conversion of glucose to glycogen for energy storage. Deficiencies in this mineral may be at the root of insulin resistance, as they throw into motion a series of interrelated imbalances at the cellular level, as I will explain in the next chapter.

Awareness of the relationship between potassium and hypertension is hardly new—it dates back to the early part of this century. A 1904 medical history published in the *Archives of General Medicine* showed that 5 out of 8 patients with hypertension successfully lowered their blood pressure by increasing their consumption of potassium-rich foods and reducing their use of table salt. Subsequent studies have supported this early work. A British study found that when 2.3 grams of potassium were administered daily to a group of patients with hypertension, blood pressure decreased by an average of 8 mm Hg. In another study, a group of African-Americans were able to reduce their blood pressure by taking a potassium supplement.

A high dietary potassium intake is also known to protect against stroke-associated deaths. In a 1998 study spearheaded by Dr. Alberto Ascherio, of Harvard Medical School, 43,738 men ages 40 to 75 were followed for eight years. It was determined that during that time, those with the lowest consumption of potassium (2.4 grams per day) had a significantly increased risk of stroke when compared with men having the highest potassium intake (4.3 grams per day). A finding of another study, conducted by Dr. Elizabeth Barrett-Connor, was even more revealing. In this study, an average daily intake of only 390 milligrams of potassium—not enough to lower blood pressure—decreased the risk of stroke by 40 percent.

▼ THE K FACTOR

Richard D. Moore, M.D., Ph.D., a researcher and professor at the State University of New York at Plattsburgh, presents a convincing case for the importance of potassium in his remarkable book *The High Blood Pressure Solution: Natural Prevention and Cure with the K Factor*. Dr. Moore has researched the potassium-hypertension connection for many years now, has an excellent grasp of the medical literature, and is a foremost expert on the subject. According to Dr. Moore, adequate potassium intake lowers blood pressure and prolongs life.

His findings show that eating foods high in potassium and low in sodium can protect against hypertension, crippling

strokes, and premature death. He goes on to demonstrate
how eating according to "K Factor" recommendations (a
potassium-to-sodium ratio of at least 4:1) can also protect
against kidney disease and reverse cardiac hypertrophy, the
abnormal growth of the heart muscle caused by hypertension. Dr. Moore maintains that increasing the proportion of
potassium to sodium in the diet protects against stroke and
premature death even if blood pressure doesn't fall. If you
want more in-depth information on the power of potassium,
his book is definitely worth reading.

HOW MUCH SODIUM?

As we have noted already, in most Americans the potassium-sodium
balance is heavily tilted in favor of sodium. Over the years, we have
developed a taste—make that a craving, in some cases—for salt. The
average American ingests about 5,000 milligrams of sodium per day,
while some consume up to 15,000 milligrams! (One teaspoon of table
salt contains about 2,000 milligrams of sodium.) When patients tell
me they haven't salted their food in years, they're surprised to learn
that most of their sodium intake may be where they least expect it—
in cereals, cookies, and even "healthy" items such as low-fat soups. At
least 80 percent of dietary sodium comes from processed foods. High
levels of sodium are found in cheeses, crackers, luncheon meats, and
virtually all canned and frozen foods. Another hidden source of
sodium is restaurant fare, from fast food to gourmet cuisine.

Federal guidelines recommend about 2,400 milligrams of sodium
per day for healthy people. Although I suggest you aim for less (under
1,000 milligrams). The real issue here is balance. According to Dr.
Moore, the ideal dietary ratio of potassium to sodium is about 4:1 for
healthy blood pressure. (For every milligram of sodium, you should
consume about 4 milligrams of potassium.) It shouldn't be hard for
you to stay within these limits if you follow the dietary recommendations I outline in Chapter 11. You'll be eating an abundance of fruits,
vegetables, and legumes—all perfectly balanced for reducing blood
pressure. Most fruits and vegetables have a potassium-to-sodium

ratio of at least 50:1, and some are much higher: bananas and oranges, for instance, at 440:1 and 260:1, respectively.

▼ | HIGH-SODIUM FOODS TO AVOID

- Frozen prepared foods
- Canned foods
- Smoked foods
- Cured foods
- Restaurant cuisine
- Most condiments
- MSG (monosodium glutamate)
- Baking soda
- Baking powder

SALT SENSITIVES, BEWARE

Some people can eat a bag of salty pretzels and their blood pressure remains normal; for others, just thinking about salt wreaks havoc with their blood pressure. An estimated 20 to 30 percent of people with hypertension have a condition called *salt sensitivity*, which means they have a severely pronounced response to sodium. Sodium restriction is extremely important for these people, as they not only have four times the risk of developing hypertension compared with people who respond normally to salt, but even small amounts of sodium can trigger a dramatic rise in blood pressure. Researchers are still looking into the mystery of salt sensitivity. Who gets it? What causes the condition? Is there a gene responsible? Although many theories exist, we still don't know for sure. Some of the possible mechanisms include kidney insufficiency, adrenal sensitivity to angiotensin, hereditary causes, or a sensitivity to the chloride fraction of salt (sodium chloride).

When I see patients who have been told they have *resistant hypertension* (abnormally high blood pressure that does not come down despite treatment with at least three drugs), I always suspect salt sensitivity. I have found that resistant hypertension can often—though not always—be remedied by strictly curtailing dietary sodium and supplementing with extra potassium. To find out if you are salt sensitive, check with your doctor or simply monitor your blood pressure response to dietary sodium changes. If you are sensitive to salt, you'll need to severely curtail your sodium intake and increase your potassium consumption.

 ## "A BANANA A DAY KEEPS THE DOCTOR AWAY"

Everybody knows that eating apples is supposed to be good for your health, but bananas? Well, according to a 1999 study, eating bananas may bring down your blood pressure. In this study, carried out at Kasturba Medical College in Manipal, India, people who ate two bananas daily for one week had a 10 percent drop in their blood pressure. In addition to containing lots of potassium, bananas may contain compounds similar to ACE inhibitors, popular drugs used to lower blood pressure.

HOW DO YOU GET THE POTASSIUM YOU NEED?

A high-potassium diet alone may give you the edge you need to overcome hypertension. Although hypertension experts currently recommend 3,400 milligrams of potassium per day, I suggest, per Dr. Moore, that you aim for the "K Factor"—the 4:1 ratio of potassium to sodium. If you eat 1,000 milligrams of sodium, then your daily intake of potassium should be at least 4,000 milligrams. It is surprisingly easy to get this much potassium in your diet: simply eat lots of fruits, vegetables, whole grains, and legumes. (A look at the list of high-potassium foods will show you how different foods stack up.) These potassium-rich foods will move your potassium-sodium ratio back into balance—and even allow you to sneak a little salt into your diet (providing that you are not salt sensitive). One thing you should be aware of is that potassium is lost when vegetables are boiled and the water discarded, so eat them raw or lightly steamed whenever possible.

▼ | HIGH-POTASSIUM FOODS

All of these foods, with the exception of fish, are very low in sodium. The potassium-to-sodium ratio in fruits and vegetables averages 50:1.

Food	Potassium (Milligrams)
Fruits	
Apple, 1 medium	182
Avocado, ½ cup	680
Banana, 1 medium	440
Cantaloupe, ¼	341
Coconut, ⅓ cup dried	588
Orange, 1 medium	263
Peach, 1 medium	308
Prunes, ⅓ cup	940
Strawberries, ½ cup	122
Vegetables and Legumes	
Asparagus, ½ cup	165
Beans	
Lima, ⅓ cup dried	1,529
Pinto, ⅓ cup dried	984
Soy, ⅓ cup dried	1,677
Cabbage, ⅓ cup raw	233
Carrot, 1 raw	225
Dulse (seaweed), ⅓ cup	8,060
Spinach, ½ cup cooked	292
Sweet potato, ⅓ cup raw	243
Tomato, 1 medium	444
Meats (3 ounces cooked)	
Chicken, light meat	350
Roast beef	224
Salmon	378
Tuna, canned, drained	225

Potassium supplements are another possibility. There are a number of good studies showing that adding potassium in supplement form to a diet can lower blood pressure by 4 to 5 mm Hg. The amount of potassium used in the studies ranged from 1,000 to 3,000 milligrams per day. However, much smaller doses are often enough, particularly if you're eating a high-potassium diet. Bob, whose story I shared on page 93, used only one to six 99-milligram tablets of potassium gluconate per day to get his blood pressure under control. In any case, I find that a healthy, plant-rich diet supplies most people with adequate potassium. Furthermore, it provides you with a host of essential vitamins and other nutrients that you won't get from potassium supplements. Another option—one we use at the Whitaker Wellness Institute and I recommend in Chapter 11—is to flavor your food with a salt substitute such as Nu-Salt, which contains potassium chloride and yields 1,056 milligrams of potassium per ¼ teaspoon.

My final suggestion comes from a salt-sensitive patient, Michael W., who found a way to solve his potassium-sodium problem. Michael had his first heart attack twenty years ago, and it severely damaged the left side of his heart. His passion for life, however, motivated him to do all he could to embrace a wellness lifestyle. His only hurdle was salt. Even a trace amount in food would cause what he called a "smothering effect," which ranged "from moderate discomfort to great peril." Then a few years ago a solution fell into his hands. Michael was introduced to something called dulse, a powdered sea vegetable with a delightfully salty taste. Michael says he can "eat a ton of it without experiencing the devastating effects of regular salt."

Though dulse tastes surprisingly salty, much of its taste comes not from sodium but from its rich mineral content. Dulse contains almost every mineral and trace mineral necessary for human health, including plenty of potassium. Although few sea vegetables are consumed by Americans, they have been eaten for centuries in Japan and Iceland. Dulse has been used in Iceland as a flavoring for almost 2,000 years, and it makes a wonderful salt substitute.

IN SUMMARY

1. Eliminate all salt-laden canned and frozen foods. Be especially careful about restaurant food. Replace table salt with a salt substitute such as Nu-Salt, NoSalt, or dulse.

2. Bring your sodium-potassium levels into balance by stepping up your potassium intake. You can do this primarily by eating potassium-rich foods, but you may want to consider taking a prescription or over-the-counter potassium supplement.

3. Get back to whole, unprocessed foods, especially fruits and vegetables, which are naturally low in sodium and high in potassium. No wholesome natural food diet has a high salt content.

4. Strive for a 4:1 ratio of potassium to sodium. You can check food labels to determine sodium content, but potassium levels are not listed. A quick look at the potassium levels in various foods in the table on page 101 shows that fruits and vegetables are generally quite high in potassium. The diet recommendations in Chapter 11 naturally provide this ratio for you.

5. Patients with kidney disease should consult their physician before adding extra potassium to their diets. Those taking potassium-sparing diuretics, ACE inhibitors, or digitalis should also check with their doctor, as potassium supplementation may be contraindicated.

CHAPTER 9

Magnesium, Calcium, and Other Beneficial Minerals

Daniel came to my clinic on the recommendation of his periodontist, who two weeks earlier had told him that his blood pressure was 240/115. It was a reality check for Daniel. Although he had a long history of hypertension and had been on blood-pressure-lowering drugs for years, because of side effects, he had simply stopped taking his medication five years earlier. At the time of his first visit, Daniel's blood pressure was 260/130. Most physicians would put a patient with blood pressure this high on medication immediately, but Daniel, who stated that he didn't like seeing physicians, was adamant about not taking drugs. He was counseled on a dietary and exercise program, started on a nutritional supplement regimen, and to quickly lower his dangerously high blood pressure, he was given a series of intravenous magnesium infusions.

Daniel's blood pressure taken before his first infusion was 210/102. After 35 minutes, it had fallen to 180/92, and after completion 15 minutes later it was 172/98. These IV drips were repeated over the next few months, each time with dramatic drops in his blood pressure. As Daniel's dietary and nutritional supplement program began to produce noticeable reductions in his blood pressure, the magnesium infusions were tapered off.

Minerals are essential for health. Without minerals your heart would stop beating, your muscles could not contract, your bones would soften, your nerves would be unable to send impulses—you literally could not live. Minerals are divided into two main groups, *macrominerals,* which are essential in larger amounts, and *microminerals,* also called trace minerals, which are necessary in minute amounts. The macrominerals are calcium, phosphorus, potassium, sulfur, sodium, chloride, and magnesium. At least eleven trace minerals are essential to human health—iron, manganese, copper, iodine, chromium, boron, molybdenum, selenium, silicon, vanadium, and zinc. Although all these minerals are important, we will cover only those most critical for healthy blood pressure.

MAGNIFICENT MAGNESIUM

Magnesium is an extremely versatile mineral. Magnesium is integral to scores of biological functions, including energy production, muscle contraction, sleep, growth, healthy pregnancy, and healing. This mineral is involved in at least 325 different enzymatic reactions, and deficiencies are known to cause seizures, psychosis, delirium, tremors, abnormal calcium deposits, and asthma. Magnesium has therapeutic effects on the cardiovascular system, and studies suggest that magnesium deficiencies may predispose individuals to elevated blood pressure and other cardiovascular conditions. Yet most Americans don't get enough of this important mineral, and deficiencies are common, particularly in the elderly. Poor diet, diuretics, diabetes, kidney disease, and dehydrating beverages such as coffee and alcohol also contribute to magnesium shortages.

▼ | MAGNESIUM-RICH FOODS

Food	Magnesium per 3½-Ounce Serving (Milligrams)
Almonds	270
Avocado	45
Brewer's yeast	231

Broccoli	24
Brown rice	88
Cashews	267
Cheddar cheese	45
Collards	57
Dulse	220
Kelp	760
Milk	13
Soybeans, cooked	88
Walnuts	131
Wheat bran	490

The initial findings establishing a link between magnesium and heart disease came from population studies data reflecting that in geographical areas where the water content of magnesium was high, hypertension and heart disease incidence were low. Inversely, low magnesium levels in the water were associated with higher rates of high blood pressure and heart disease. In one study, the risk for hypertension was found to be 3.61 times greater in regions with lower magnesium concentrations in the drinking water. This and similar observations led scientists to consider the role of magnesium in cardiovascular health and to pursue more in-depth studies on the mineral.

The Atherosclerosis Risk in Communities (ARIC) Study, published in the July 1995 issue of the *Journal of Clinical Epidemiology*, examined the relationships between serum and dietary magnesium and cardiovascular disease. It was discovered that magnesium levels were significantly lower in study participants with hypertension, diabetes, and heart disease than in participants with normal blood pressure and blood sugar levels and no history of heart disease. The earlier Honolulu Heart Study showed this inverse relationship to be true as well. Systolic blood pressure was 6.4 mm Hg lower and diastolic was 3.1 mm Hg lower in the group with the highest magnesium intake, compared with the group consuming the least magnesium.

Magnesium affects blood pressure in several ways. Low levels of this mineral are associated with increased activity of renin, the RAAS enzyme that contributes to hypertension. Magnesium is also required for the proper working of the sodium-potassium pump and sodium battery described in the previous chapter. These cellular processes fuel the calcium pump, which helps regulate blood pressure. Most important, magnesium acts as a vasodilator—it relaxes and dilates the arteries, allowing the blood to flow more freely, exerting less resistance on the "pipes" and bringing down blood pressure. Magnesium does this by controlling the access of calcium into arterial cells, most likely by stabilizing cellular membranes. As I've explained in previous chapters, excess calcium inside the cells (not circulating in the blood) increases muscle tension, peripheral resistance, and blood pressure.

Because it prevents excess calcium from entering cells, much as calcium channel blockers do, magnesium has been called nature's calcium channel blocker. However, unlike the synthetic drugs, magnesium is nontoxic and inexpensive and has many other health benefits. Although I use intravenous magnesium in my clinic with patients like Daniel to bring down dangerously elevated blood pressure, taking oral magnesium supplements to help keep blood pressure under control clearly works, as has been demonstrated in several well-designed studies. In one double-blind, placebo-controlled study, 91 middle-aged women with mild to moderate hypertension, not treated with drugs, were divided into two groups. One group was administered daily magnesium supplements, while the other group received a placebo. After six months, both the systolic and diastolic blood pressures of the magnesium group dropped an average of 2.7 mm Hg. There was little or no change in the placebo group. In another study, 18 diuretic-dependent hypertensive patients who were deficient in magnesium (a common deficiency in patients on diuretics) were given daily magnesium supplements and experienced an average blood pressure drop of 8 mm Hg.

MAGNESIUM PROTECTS AGAINST INSULIN RESISTANCE

Magnesium is also one of the most important minerals for the prevention and reversal of insulin resistance, which is an underlying cause of hypertension. According to Dr. Lawrence Resnik, of Cornell University, insulin resistance is caused at least in part by a defect at the cellular level in the regulation of magnesium and calcium. Magnesium improves insulin sensitivity, while intracellular calcium impedes these processes. A 1993 study published in the *Indian Journal of Medical Science* demonstrated that low magnesium levels were associated with high blood glucose, indicating an insulin-resistant state. However, when high magnesium concentrations were present in the blood, circulating glucose levels were lower, suggesting that magnesium was instrumental in helping usher glucose into the cells.

Supplemental magnesium can do much to counter insulin resistance. By improving insulin sensitivity and glucose uptake by the cells, therapeutic dosages of magnesium can help put the brakes on insulin resistance. Magnesium supplementation is crucial for anyone with hypertension, insulin resistance, or any of the manifestations of syndrome X (see page 62). I recommend taking 1,000 milligrams of magnesium every day.

CALCIUM, HYPERTENSION, AND INSULIN RESISTANCE

Calcium is the most abundant mineral in the human body and comprises about 2 percent of your total body weight. It helps regulate the heartbeat and is the major mineral required for healthy bones, strong teeth, muscle contractions, blood clotting, and the release of important neurotransmitters. Sometimes called magnesium's "second cousin," calcium is intimately related to magnesium at the cellular level. Adequate blood levels of calcium are also necessary for normal sodium-potassium balance, and it is instrumental in both blood pressure regulation and insulin utilization.

As I described briefly in the previous chapter, the sodium battery (which is charged up by the sodium-potassium pump) drives the calcium pump, which pumps excess calcium out of the cells. Too much calcium in the smooth muscle cells of the arteries causes them to tense up or contract, resulting in increased peripheral resistance in the arteries and elevations in blood pressure. Calcium is also a factor in insulin resistance. High levels of intracellular calcium decrease the ability of the cells to usher in glucose in the presence of insulin. Therefore, glucose and insulin build up in the bloodstream.

Paradoxical as this may seem at first glance, adequate calcium levels in the body keep excess calcium from entering the cells, and low levels cause a buildup inside the cells. The pressure exerted by extracellular calcium on the cellular membrane keeps it healthy and prevents leakiness that allows excess calcium to get in. This results in less tension in the blood vessels and healthy blood pressure. Although the data supporting the use of calcium supplementation in the treatment of hypertension isn't always consistent, there are a few clinical trials demonstrating that calcium effects a reduction in blood pressure.

In a study published in the 1991 *American Journal of Hypertension,* twenty-four-hour ambulatory blood pressure monitors (ABPM) were used in a group of elderly patients to study the effects of calcium supplementation on mild to moderate hypertension. When these study subjects took 1,000 milligrams of calcium daily, they experienced an average decline in blood pressure of 13.6 mm Hg systolic and 5.0 mm Hg diastolic. Another study, a six-month trial conducted by Cornell University Medical School researchers, demonstrated that 2 grams of calcium carbonate daily in four divided doses resulted in a "modest but consistent fall" in blood pressure in 26 patients. Average blood pressure in these subjects fell from 161/94 to 154/89—and some participants experienced a 10 to 20 percent reduction in diastolic blood pressure. Supplemental calcium's beneficial effects on blood pressure have been confirmed in a number of more recent studies, although the declines in blood pressure have been less dramatic.

To ensure adequate calcium intake, I recommend that you include calcium-rich foods in your diet (many of the same foods that contain potassium and magnesium are also high in calcium) and supplement with 1,000 milligrams of calcium per day.

▼ CALCIUM-RICH FOODS

Food	Calcium per 3½-Ounce Serving (Milligrams)
Almonds	234
Beans, dry, cooked	50
Brewer's yeast	210
Cheddar cheese	750
Collard greens	250
Cottage cheese	94
Kale	249
Kelp	1,093
Milk	118
Parsley	203
Sesame seeds	110
Soybeans, cooked	73
Sunflower seeds	120
Yogurt	120

TRACE MINERALS AGAINST HYPERTENSION

The body also requires certain microminerals for healthy blood pressure. In fact, big problems can arise from tiny deficiencies of these nutrients. Let's take a look at the trace minerals most important for blood pressure control and insulin sensitivity.

Chromium

Chromium is a critical component of glucose tolerance factor (GTF), which improves the action of insulin and facilitates the uptake of glucose into the cells. Many of the studies examining chromium's effects on insulin and resistance have involved patients with type II diabetes. Deficiencies of chromium are common in this condition, and supplementation generally results in improvements in fasting glucose levels, glucose tolerance, and insulin levels, as well as cholesterol and triglyceride levels. Although little research has been done on chromium's direct effects on blood pressure, because it markedly improves insulin sensitivity this mineral is a valuable therapy for patients with hypertension associated with insulin resistance.

Chromium also facilitates weight loss and at the same time increases lean body (muscle) mass, thus improving body mass index (BMI) and reducing the risk of hypertension. This was demonstrated in a 1998 study conducted by Dr. Gilbert R. Kaats and colleagues of the Health and Medical Research Foundation in San Antonio. One hundred twenty-two subjects were given 400 micrograms of chromium picolinate per day or placebo, while their diets and exercise regimens were monitored. After ninety days, adjusting for caloric intake and expenditure, it was determined that chromium did indeed have positive effects on weight and body composition. The individuals taking chromium lost more weight (an average of 17.1 pounds compared with 3.9 pounds for the placebo group), fat mass (16.9 pounds versus 3.3 pounds), and percentage of body fat (6.3 percent versus 1.2 percent).

Concerns have been raised in recent years about the safety of chromium. However, numerous animal and human studies have demonstrated that chromium is extremely safe. In one toxicity study, rats fed the human equivalent of thousands of 200-microgram tablets showed no signs of toxicity. The Ames test, commonly used to identify potential cancer-causing substances, also gave chromium the thumbs-up.

Whole grains, meats, and brewer's yeast are the most abundant food sources of this important mineral. Several types of chromium supplements are available, but the best-absorbed forms are chromium picolinate and chromium polynicotinate. I suggest a dosage of 200 micrograms of chromium per day for best results.

Vanadium

Vanadium is another trace element with very promising effects on insulin resistance. It improves insulin sensitivity and even appears to act as an insulin "mimic" by activating insulin receptors on the cells and facilitating the entry of glucose into cells. In fact, research conducted in the mid-1990s by John McNeill, Ph.D., at the University of British Columbia in Vancouver, has demonstrated that sufficient doses of vanadyl sulfate (one form of the mineral) completely reversed type II diabetes in laboratory animals and its effect lasted even after the supplement was discontinued. Other studies have verified the therapeutic benefits of vanadyl sulfate in the treatment of human diabetes as well. Dr. McNeill has also studied the effects of vanadium on hypertension. He fed laboratory animals large amounts of fructose, which caused high blood pressure and increased insulin levels. He then gave the animals vanadium and found that this caused "marked and sustained decreases in plasma insulin concentration and blood pressure."

Some of the best food sources of vanadium are whole grains, soybeans, shellfish, mushrooms, dill, and parsley. Considering the close relationship between hypertension and insulin resistance, I believe that vanadium supplementation could dramatically benefit many patients with hypertension. If you choose to give vanadyl sulfate a trial on your own, take no more than 45 milligrams per day, in divided doses. This should be enough for most individuals with hypertension. However, more is often required for vanadium to demonstrate its insulin-like effects, and I recommend 100 to 150 milligrams for individuals who also have severe insulin resistance or type II diabetes. However, vanadium in these higher doses should only be taken under the direction of a physician, as it may result in dramatic declines in blood sugar.

Other Trace Minerals

We have discussed the minerals most intimately involved in the regulation and treatment of hypertension. It is likely, however, that others are involved in supporting roles. Zinc, for example, is one of the most important of the trace minerals, and its functions in the body are widespread. Deficiencies in this mineral are linked to several disorders, including impaired glucose tolerance and obesity. Zinc's relationship to copper is particularly critical, and imbalances between the two—too much copper and not enough zinc—are not uncommon in hypertension. This can be corrected by simply increas-

ing your zinc intake. Since this mineral is also critical for insulin production, I recommend zinc supplementation to all of my overweight,
diabetic, and hypertensive patients. An effective dose is 30 milligrams
daily.

Another mineral that may be involved in hypertension is selenium.
Selenium is a very powerful antioxidant, and research shows that
when levels of this mineral are low, risk of cardiovascular disease, premature aging, and cancer goes up. It also counters the toxic effects of
heavy metals including lead, mercury, aluminum, and cadmium,
which have been implicated in hypertension. Although most of the
research on selenium has examined its relationship to cancer and
heart disease, a few studies have suggested that low blood levels of selenium might be a risk factor for the development of hypertension.
While you can get this important mineral from selected foods (especially whole grains), the selenium content in food is in direct proportion to the amount that's in the soil—which means there's no
guarantee as to how much you're getting. For this reason I recommend taking a selenium supplement of 200 micrograms per day. The
best-absorbed form is high-yeast selenium.

Nutritional science is a rapidly expanding field. I have no doubt
that in future years the importance of other minerals and nutritional
elements in the development and treatment of hypertension and insulin resistance will be uncovered. Your best bet is to take a multivitamin and mineral supplement that contains an array of macro- and
microminerals.

IN SUMMARY

1. Add mineral-rich foods to your diet. I've listed some good suggestions in this chapter.
2. Take a broad-spectrum multiple vitamin and mineral supplement (as described in the next chapter), plus enough additional
   magnesium to total an average of 1,000 milligrams per day. For
   example, if your multivitamin contains 500 milligrams of magnesium, you would need to add 500 milligrams from a supple-

mental magnesium source such as magnesium citrate, magnesium ascorbate, or magnesium gluconate.

3. Balance your magnesium with a good calcium supplement so you get at least equal amounts of both minerals (1,000 milligrams magnesium, 1,000 milligrams calcium). Good sources of calcium include calcium gluconate, calcium ascorbate, calcium citrate, and calcium malate.

4. Take 200 micrograms of chromium picolinate or chromium polynicotinate and 45 to 150 milligrams vanadyl sulfate (100 milligrams or more should only be taken under the close supervision of a physician). You will probably need to supplement these separately, as most multivitamin and mineral formulas don't contain adequate amounts—if any—of these minerals.

5. Make sure your multivitamin and mineral formula contains 30 milligrams of zinc and 200 micrograms of selenium.

CHAPTER 10

Nutritional Supplements Against Hypertension

Jean was diagnosed with high blood pressure ten years ago and was immediately prescribed a low-dose beta-blocker. For the next ten years her blood pressure remained under good control, but she was bothered by side effects of her medication. She felt constantly tired, her hands and feet were always cold, and she noticed occasional numbness and tingling in her fingers. As her symptoms worsened over the years, Jean started exploring alternatives to the blood pressure drugs she had been told she would require for the rest of her life. Convinced that there was a better, safer way to manage her blood pressure, Jean enrolled in the weeklong program at the Whitaker Wellness Institute two years ago.

I started Jean on a comprehensive nutritional supplement program of vitamins, minerals, essential fatty acids, herbs, and coenzyme Q10. At the same time, as part of the program at the Institute, she was exercising daily, eating a diet designed to lower blood pressure, drinking a lot of water, and participating in stress management classes. We decided to discontinue her medication for the week and observe her blood pressure. Although she was somewhat leery of this—after all, she had been told she would have to take this medication for the rest of her life—her blood pressure remained in the normal range. Jean left the Institute with recommendations to continue on her nutritional supplements, diet, and exercise and stress management programs. Because her blood pressure had responded so beautifully to these lifestyle changes, she was advised to stay off her medication, continue monitoring her blood pressure, and let me know if it began to creep up. Much to Jean's surprise and delight, her pressure has remained in the normal range for two years now. The circulation in her hands and feet has improved, and she feels more energetic than she has in years.

I believe that the single most important thing you can do for your overall health is to take nutritional supplements. This is not a statement I make lightly. Since I veered away from conventional medicine more than twenty-five years ago, I've used a three-pronged treatment approach: diet, exercise, and nutritional supplementation. I initially assumed that diet and exercise were the most powerful of these tools. As I told you in the introduction to this book, I had seen seriously ill people get well simply by changing their diets. However, with the volumes of research that have emerged in the last fifty years demonstrating the incredible benefits of vitamins, minerals, essential fatty acids, amino acids, botanicals, and other natural substances, I've become convinced that nutritional supplements are the most powerful tools in medicine today. And I believe that if every physician were open-minded enough to utilize these safe, effective therapies—not to the exclusion of conventional drugs and surgery, but as an adjunct—our nation's health would improve tremendously.

A study published in the *Western Journal of Medicine* in 1997 examined the potential benefits of just three nutritional supplements: vitamin E, folic acid, and zinc. The researchers calculated that if every American in targeted groups took these supplements, there would be a net reduction in health care costs of almost $20 billion per year. According to this study, if everyone over 50 years of age took vitamin E, hospital costs associated with heart disease would be reduced by 38 percent. If women of childbearing age took folic acid, the hospital costs of caring for children born with neural tube birth defects would be lowered by 40 percent, and if these same women took zinc, the costs of caring for low-birth-weight babies would drop by 60 percent. Imagine, a savings of $20 billion simply by taking three supplements! And just think about the human suffering that would be avoided.

Don't underestimate the power of targeted nutritional supplements. If the systems in your body involved in regulating blood pressure, beginning at the cellular level, do not receive the raw materials they need to function and regenerate, the entire works go awry. As I've stated before, hypertension is caused in part by deficiencies and imbalances of certain nutrients. One of the very first steps you should take toward lowering your blood pressure is to implement the suggestions for supplementation I've made in this book. It is a cornerstone of this program for reversing hypertension.

WHO NEEDS NUTRITIONAL SUPPLEMENTS?

Virtually everyone needs nutritional supplements. So much of the food we eat is stripped of nutrients that even if you eat a very healthy diet—which few people do—you cannot be assured that your food has all the nutritional value you would expect. In addition, a number of other factors can rob your body of the nutrients it so desperately needs to function optimally. Environmental and lifestyle stressors increase your nutrient needs beyond what even the healthiest diet can provide. Smokers, for example, have been found to have low levels of vitamins C, E, and beta-carotene—up to 30 percent lower than nonsmokers. And the elderly frequently have nutritional deficiencies due to decreased caloric intake, poor nutrient absorption, and long-term prescription drug use.

▼ | FACTORS THAT ROB YOUR BODY OF NUTRIENTS

- Poor diet
- Regular caffeine intake
- Regular alcohol consumption
- Chronic dieting
- Prescription or over-the-counter drugs
- Infection or illness
- Chronic stress
- Pregnancy
- Diabetes and other diseases

- Cigarette smoke
- Aging
- Poor digestion
- Injury, trauma, or surgery
- Exposure to pollutants

The best dietary sources of important vitamins and minerals are plant foods. Unfortunately, only 9 percent of the American population eat the recommended five daily servings of fruits and vegetables. In fact, a survey of 11,658 people conducted by the U.S. Department of Agriculture came up with some startling figures. On an average day 41 percent of Americans eat no fruit, 72 percent consume no vitamin C-rich fruits, 82 percent have no cruciferous vegetables (broccoli, cabbage, etc.), and 84 percent eat no high-fiber, whole-grain foods. With dietary habits like these, is it any wonder that we are riddled with degenerative diseases? Furthermore, at least 70 percent of the food most of us eat has been processed. Processed foods are stripped of fiber. Their natural, healthy oils have been altered by chemicals and heat, resulting in the creation of harmful free radicals and trans fatty acids. And their vitamin and mineral content is severely depleted.

The sad truth is that even if you do eat a healthy diet rich in plant foods, you cannot be assured of getting optimal nutrition. The nutrient content of plant foods is dependent upon the quality of the soil in which the foods were grown: if the soils are deficient in certain minerals, the plants will be similarly deficient. Storage is another factor that affects the nutritional value of food. The longer vegetables and fruits are stored, the more significant the nutrient losses, and some of them—apples and root vegetables such as potatoes, for example—are routinely stored for months on end. Frozen foods also lose nutrients if they are partially defrosted and refrozen during shipping or storage.

I strongly feel that everyone should take a good multivitamin and mineral supplement on a daily basis. It's like an insurance policy against the harmful effects of a poor diet—and the unknowns in a decent diet. The older you are, the more important taking nutritional supplements becomes. As we age, our digestive system becomes less efficient at extracting nutrients from food, and there are many studies demonstrating that nutrient levels in older people are lower than in younger people. The resultant deficiencies put us at increased risk of degenerative disease.

It is clear that dietary imbalances are a major contributor to high blood pressure, atherosclerosis, and other degenerative diseases. The Public Health Service claims that dietary and nutritional factors are implicated in four of the ten leading causes of death in the United States—cardiovascular disease, cancer, stroke, and diabetes—and notes that these illnesses represent two-thirds of all deaths. With this in mind, I believe everybody should take extra steps to ensure that their nutritional needs are met. In the previous chapter we discussed the minerals involved in blood pressure control. In this chapter we will cover other vital nutritional supplements for preventing and reversing hypertension: antioxidants, B-complex vitamins, omega-3 fatty acids, coenzyme Q10, arginine, garlic, and hawthorn.

HOW FREE RADICALS AFFECT BLOOD PRESSURE

Free radicals are unstable molecules that attempt to stabilize themselves by stealing electrons from healthy cells. This damages the previously healthy cells, which then become highly unstable themselves and steal electrons from other cells, creating a chain reaction of cellular destruction. Free radicals are a natural by-product of cellular metabolism—they are produced as cells extract energy from food in the presence of oxygen. However, their production is further accelerated by exposure to cigarette smoke and other toxins, ultraviolet radiation from the sun, and dietary factors, such as rancid fats. The cellular injury caused by free radicals is called *oxidative stress* or *oxidative damage,* and it is the dominant theory of why we age.

It is also a key factor in hypertension, primarily because it contributes to atherosclerosis and arteriosclerosis. The atherosclerotic process begins with injury to the endothelial cells lining the arterial wall. This may be caused by an infectious agent, a chemical toxin, impairments in the activity of nitric oxide, or the physical pounding that results from elevated blood pressure. Small blood cells called platelets and larger white blood cells called monocytes adhere to the injured area and initiate the abnormal growth of smooth muscle cells and the buildup of oxidized LDL cholesterol and white blood cells called macrophages and changed into foam cells, which burrow into the artery wall.

As the arteries become narrowed by these deposits, blood flow is impeded and blood pressure is increased. The arteries begin to harden and become less elastic, losing their ability to dilate and constrict on cue. Eventually they become unresponsive to the body's internal messages to regulate blood pressure which are conveyed by nerve impulses, hormones, and other chemicals. One of the most powerful of these chemical messengers, nitric oxide (a vasodilator that, as discussed in Chapter 2, relaxes arteries and lowers blood pressure), is inactivated by excessive amounts of oxidized LDL cholesterol. This is yet another way in which free radical damage contributes to hypertension.

Higher than average levels of lipid peroxidation (free radical damage to fatty tissues) and imbalances in antioxidant status have been observed in patients with hypertension. In a 1998 study published in the *Journal of Hypertension,* Italian researchers compared oxidation and antioxidant balances in 105 patients recently diagnosed with hypertension and 100 people with normal blood pressure. They found that subjects with high blood pressure had impairments in antioxidant status, an increased response to oxidative stress, or both. Impairments were seen in the activity of vitamin E and vitamin A, two antioxidants that, as you will see below, work in the lipid (fatty) tissues of the body to help prevent the oxidation of LDL cholesterol. Other studies have demonstrated similar results, with lower levels of and reduced protection from vitamin C in hypertensives as well. These deficiencies may contribute to the tendency of patients with hypertension to develop atherosclerosis.

ANTIOXIDANTS FOR YOUR
CARDIOVASCULAR SYSTEM

Free radical production is as inevitable as breathing and eating, but nature has provided us with an antidote that counteracts oxidative damage caused by free radicals: *antioxidants*. Antioxidants neutralize highly reactive free radicals by giving them electrons, thus ending their chain reaction of destruction and protecting healthy cells from damage. The antioxidant vitamins C, E, A, and beta-carotene are the major free radical fighters against hypertension and heart disease.

Vitamin C

Vitamin C protects your arteries and decreases the risk of heart disease and hypertension in several ways. First, vitamin C prevents the generation of free radicals, which are believed to contribute to atherosclerosis by damaging artery walls. Second, it helps repair damage to the arteries, preventing the deposit of plaque at the site of injury. It also strengthens and restores the elasticity of the blood vessels and improves vasodilation by restoring nitric oxide activity. And finally, vitamin C elevates levels of HDL cholesterol, the type of cholesterol that protects against atherosclerosis (as opposed to LDL cholesterol, which contributes to blockages).

The late two-time Nobel laureate Linus Pauling, Ph.D., contended for years that chronically low levels of vitamin C (ascorbic acid) promote atherosclerosis. Dr. Pauling, together with Matthias Rath, M.D., convincingly demonstrated that the primary cause of arterial blockages may not be LDL cholesterol but a particle that resembles LDL cholesterol called lipoprotein a, or Lp(a). Lp(a) has a small strand of protein attached to it that adheres to damaged areas on the artery walls, initiating the buildup of plaque. However, because vitamin C is also attracted to these damaged areas and works quickly to facilitate artery repair, adequate vitamin C levels ensure that Lp(a) won't be able to do its damage. Most mammals produce vitamin C in the liver. However, the dangerous Lp(a) particle is found primarily in mammals that do not make vitamin C: humans and other primates, guinea pigs, and one species of bats. Drs. Pauling and Rath maintained that atherosclerosis is likely caused by a vitamin C deficiency that is worsened by other risk factors—such as a high-fat diet or smoking—that further deplete the body of vitamin C. They concluded: "It will be hard for any pharmaceutical product to surpass ascorbate [a form of vitamin C], a substance that has been developed by nature over billions of years."

Others have confirmed vitamin C's protective effects on the cardiovascular system. Dr. Ishwarlal Jialal, winner of the American Heart Association's 1989 Young Investigator Award, compared the ability of vitamin C, vitamin E, and beta-carotene to block cholesterol buildup in the arteries. Vitamin E was 45 percent effective and beta-carotene was 90 percent effective, but the most powerful protector was vitamin C, which was an astounding 95 percent effective!

Vitamin C also lowers the risk of death from cardiovascular disease. Dr. James Engstrom, associate professor at UCLA School of Public Health, conducted a survey of 11,348 men and women and found that men with the highest intake of vitamin C had a 45 percent lower risk of death from heart disease compared with those having the lowest intake of vitamin C. Women in the high-intake group had a 25 percent reduced risk compared with those in the lowest group.

Several studies have found that blood levels of vitamin C are significantly lower in patients with high blood pressure than in those with normal blood pressure. In a recent nutritional survey of nearly 1,000 British citizens over 65 years of age, low intakes of vitamin C were consistently associated with elevated blood pressure. In fact, vitamin C was the only nutrient noted in this study to have an inverse relationship with blood pressure. The government-mandated recommended daily allowance (RDA) of vitamin C is an absurdly low 60 milligrams per day. If you have hypertension, I recommend a minimum of 2,500 milligrams of vitamin C per day.

Vitamin E

Vitamin E is the most active antioxidant in the fatty cells of your body, as it breaks the chain of lipid peroxidation that destroys cell membranes and other fat-containing tissues. Vitamin E reduces the risk of heart disease and hypertension by protecting your arteries from the devastating effects of oxidized LDL cholesterol, which is a primary factor in the genesis of atherosclerosis and hypertension, as it inhibits the production of nitric oxide. The powerful effects of this nutrient against heart disease made national news as early as June 10,

1946, when *Time* magazine reported the findings of Drs. Evan and Wilfrid Shute of London, Ontario. The magazine hailed the researchers' work on vitamin E as "a startling discovery: a treatment for heart disease (the nation's No. 1 killer) which so far has succeeded against all common forms of the ailment. . . . Large concentrated doses of vitamin E . . . benefited four types of heart ailment (95% of the total): arteriosclerotic, hypertensive, rheumatic, old and new coronary heart disease. The vitamin helped a failing heart. It eliminated anginal pain."

I am amazed that so many physicians continue to ignore this important nutrient. Can you imagine how many lives might have been saved over the last fifty years if more physicians and their patients had embraced this humble vitamin? In the fifty-plus years since the Shute brothers published their groundbreaking work, a strong and growing body of research has confirmed the value of vitamin E in protecting against heart disease. Among the more recent studies demonstrating the protective powers of this inexpensive vitamin were those carried out at Harvard University and published in the *New England Journal of Medicine.* In one of these studies, 87,245 female nurses were closely followed for eight years. Their vitamin E intake was monitored, and the incidence of heart attack and death from heart disease was recorded. Researchers found that the nurses who took at least 100 international units of vitamin E daily for more than two years had a 41 percent lower risk of heart disease than nonusers of the vitamin. A second study involved 39,910 male physicians who were followed for a similar period of time. It was discovered that the men who had a daily intake of more than 30 international units of vitamin E had a 37 percent reduction in heart disease.

Controlled clinical trials of the value of vitamin E supplements have also been conducted. The Cambridge Heart Antioxidant Study (CHAOS) was a double-blind, placebo-controlled study that involved 2,002 patients with coronary heart disease. Study subjects were divided into two groups, and one group was given 400 to 800 international units of vitamin E daily in supplement form, while the other group received placebo pills. After an average of 510 days, the patients taking vitamin E had 75 percent fewer heart attacks than the placebo group. Although this and other studies have focused on prevention of heart attacks, don't forget that the number one *cause* of heart attacks is atherosclerosis, which is also a causative factor in hypertension.

For the treatment and prevention of hypertension, I recommend taking 800 international units of natural vitamin E daily. Make sure your supplement contains natural vitamin E (indicated on the label as d-alpha-tocopheryl or d-alpha-tocopherol), preferably with mixed tocopherols (other forms of natural vitamin E). Synthetic vitamin E (*dl*-alpha-tocopheryl or *dl*-alpha-tocopherol) is a poor substitute.

Vitamin A and Beta-Carotene

Vitamin A is a fat-soluble vitamin that, like vitamin E, works primarily in the lipid, or fat, tissues of your body. Although it appears to be less powerful than vitamin E in protecting against damage to the arteries, vitamin A is capable of neutralizing highly reactive oxygen free radicals. It does this by absorbing the destructive energy of these particles into its own molecular structures and slowly discharging this energy in a safe manner.

Vitamin A also prevents LDL cholesterol from being oxidized by free radicals. Remember, it is the oxidation of LDL cholesterol—not cholesterol itself—that promotes the buildup of plaque in your arteries. In a major study conducted by the World Health Organization (WHO), involving thousands of men and women from sixteen different countries, low levels of vitamin A and vitamin E in the blood were more than twice as predictive of a heart attack than either elevated blood cholesterol levels or elevated blood pressure. In participants who possessed all four risk factors—low vitamin E, low vitamin A, high blood cholesterol, and high blood pressure—the risk of heart attack was an alarming 87 percent.

Beta-carotene, which is often referred to as "pro-vitamin A," is a naturally occurring antioxidant that is readily metabolized in the liver into vitamin A. Vitamin A can be toxic in very high doses, but beta-carotene is extremely safe. I routinely recommend both vitamin A and beta-carotene in daily doses of 5,000 and 15,000 international units, respectively, to protect against cardiovascular disease. While I am well aware of the toxicity issues surrounding vitamin A use, I feel they are overblown. In my own practice, I have never observed any vitamin A toxicity with doses of 5,000 to 10,000 international units per day, and I routinely prescribe short courses of even higher doses to treat infections. However, because some studies have shown a weak link between birth defects and dosages above 10,000 international units per day during pregnancy, I recommend that women who are pregnant or might get pregnant not exceed this dose. Beta-carotene may be taken in doses greater than 15,000 international units with no fear of toxicity.

B-COMPLEX VITAMINS:
POWER AGAINST HYPERTENSION

As you've begun to realize, atherosclerosis is more than a simple matter of cholesterol sticking to arterial walls. Other factors are involved, and chief among these is *homocysteine*. Homocysteine is a toxic by-product of an essential chemical reaction that occurs during the digestion and breakdown of protein. While homocysteine is extremely toxic to the body, it is normally converted into the harmless amino acid methionine with the help of folic acid and vitamin B-12, or into cysteine, another amino acid, with the assistance of vitamin B-6. This process is called *methylation*, and it is in a sense your body's house-cleaning mechanism. By detoxifying homocysteine, methylation helps protect against atherosclerosis, cancer, and dementia.

If you are deficient in these B vitamins, however, homocysteine builds up inside your cells and eventually spills into the bloodstream, stimulating the production of a highly reactive form of homocysteine called homocysteine thiolactone. This toxic compound interferes with oxygen utilization and results in the formation of free radicals that harm the lining of the arteries. It also encourages the formation of blood clots, stimulates the growth of excess muscle tissue in the arterial walls, and allows LDL cholesterol to be more easily deposited.

The early research on homocysteine conducted by pioneering Harvard medical researcher Kilmer S. McCully, M.D., in the late 1960s was ridiculed by his colleagues, and he was eventually asked to leave Harvard. In recent years, however, Dr. McCully has been vindicated, as hundreds of articles in medical journals have confirmed the relationship between atherosclerosis, elevated homocysteine levels, and low intakes of vitamin B-6, vitamin B-12, and folic acid. A 1996 study found that individuals with higher homocysteine levels had low levels of folic acid and vitamin B-6, along with substantially increased blockages of their carotid arteries. Blockages in these major arteries to the brain are strongly linked to the incidence of stroke. Perhaps the most conclusive study of the connection between homocysteine and cardiovascular disease was an investigation published in the June 11, 1997, issue of the *New England Journal of Medicine*. The authors of the study concluded, "An increased plasma total homocysteine level confers an independent risk of vascular disease similar to that of smoking or hyperlipidemia [elevated cholesterol and/or triglycerides]. It powerfully increases the risk associated with smoking and hypertension."

At the same time, it has also been shown that higher intakes of folic acid and vitamin B-6 protect against heart disease. A 1998 Harvard survey of more than 80,000 women found that after adjustments were made for all other risk factors, the women with the highest intakes of folate (the form of folic acid found in food) and vitamin B-6 had a 45 percent decrease in the risk of heart attack. Furthermore, the women with the lowest incidence of heart attack had average intakes of 700 micrograms of folic acid and 5.6 milligrams of vitamin B-6 per day— levels much higher than the current RDAs.

Several studies of different population groups have also found a direct link between elevated homocysteine and high blood pressure. In a 1997 *Circulation* study, elevated homocysteine levels were shown to be an independent risk factor for hypertension in older people. Yet a large-scale study conducted in Hordaland County in western Norway found that among individuals with no serious history of disease, elevated homocysteine levels were associated with high blood pressure and other risk factors for cardiovascular disease. Another study demonstrated links between high homocysteine levels and elevated diastolic blood pressure in patients with type II diabetes. Type II diabetes, as you recall from Chapter 6, is caused by severe insulin resistance, itself a player in hypertension.

Given the overwhelming evidence of the harmful effects of homocysteine—and the power of B-complex vitamins to render this toxin harmless—I recommend daily supplementation of B-complex vitamins, especially folic acid (800 micrograms), vitamin B-12 (100 micrograms), and vitamin B-6 (75 milligrams). Vitamin B-6 also has independent blood-pressure-lowering effects. In a 1995 study, twenty patients with hypertension were administered daily B-6 supplements for four weeks. Decreases were observed in their levels of normal epinephrine—a blood-borne chemical that elevates blood pressure by causing the arteries to constrict and the heart to beat with more force. This was accompanied by average decreases in systolic pressure from 167 to 153 and in diastolic from 108 to 98.

ESSENTIAL FATTY ACIDS HELP NORMALIZE BLOOD PRESSURE

Just as a car needs the right kind of oil to keep running smoothly, your body needs the right kinds of fats. Although fats are generally scorned in discussions of health, certain fats are required for the optimal functioning of the human body. Essential fatty acids (EFAs) have a unique chemical structure that makes them metabolically active and able to perform functions that no other fats can. They energize your circulatory, digestive, immune and nervous systems, and create robust cell membranes.

There are two types of EFAs, classified as omega-3 and omega-6 fatty acids. Our diet contains ample omega-6 fatty acids, which are found in nuts, grains, and vegetable oils. We are likely to be deficient, however, in the omega-3 fatty acids, which are found primarily in cold-water fish such as salmon and mackerel and also in flaxseed. Yet it is the omega-3s that offer the most potent protection against hypertension. They are converted into docosahexanoic acid (DHA) as well as eicosapentaenoic acid (EPA), the precursor to powerful prostaglandins—hormonelike chemical messengers that help regulate blood pressure.

To better understand how omega-3 fatty acids can prevent and treat hypertension, let's consider their role in five different areas of cardiovascular health. As you look at this list, think about how, according to the pump-pipes model of hypertension, these factors influence blood pressure.

Blood fats: Omega-3 fatty acids can have a marked effect on reducing cholesterol and triglyceride levels. Researchers at the University of Oregon found that in just four weeks on a diet high in fish oils, 10 patients with markedly high triglycerides (1,353 mg/dl) experienced a drop to 281 mg/dl, while their cholesterol fell from 373 to 207 mg/dl. I regularly see similar improvements in my patients.

Clotting factor: One of the major cardiovascular benefits of increasing omega-3 fatty acids in your diet is the effect they have on your blood's coagulability, or tendency to clot. An abnormal blood clot in a partially blocked artery often initiates a heart attack. Omega-3 fatty acids reduce the production of a dangerous substance known as thromboxane A2 that stimulates abnormal blood clotting and thus decreases the risk of heart attacks and strokes. Ten capsules of fish oil per day have been demonstrated to not only reduce the production of thromboxane A2, but also increase the synthesis of a natural blood thinner.

Blood flow: When omega-3 oils are consumed, there is a rapid uptake of fatty acids by both the blood platelets (which are necessary for blood clotting) and the red blood cells. This action measurably reduces the tendency of the platelets to clump together and initiate a clot, while making the red blood cells more flexible and substantially improving blood flow through the small capillaries.

Blood pressure: Not surprisingly, if the blood is less viscous and flows more freely, resistance on the artery walls decreases, allowing blood pressure to fall. Over 60 double-blind studies in which fish oils were administered to hypertensive patients observed that blood pressure did indeed fall with supplemental omega-3 fatty acids.

Atherosclerosis: Omega-3 fatty acids also help prevent atherosclerosis. In a study conducted on pigs fed a diet high in saturated fat and cholesterol, half of the pigs received 30 milliliters of cod-liver oil per day while the other half (the control group) did not. When the animals were autopsied eight months later, the coronary arteries in the control group had obvious and substantial clogging. In the group receiving 30 milliliters of cod-liver oil, however, there was almost no atherosclerosis. This protective effect occurred even though the blood cholesterol and blood fat levels in both groups were essentially the same.

According to Harvard's Alexander Leaf, M.D., one of the foremost experts on EFAs, our hunter-gatherer ancestors consumed a 1:5 or 1:6 ratio of omega-3 fatty acids to omega-6 fatty acids. (Other experts estimate the ratio to be as much as 1:1.) Game animals that consume substantial amounts of green vegetables have far more omega-3 fatty acids in their flesh and body oils than do grain-fed feedlot animals, which are virtually void of these fats. The ratio of omega-3 fatty acids to omega-6 fatty acids in today's westernized diet is between 1:20 and 1:30, and that, my friends, is dangerous. By immediately and substantially increasing your intake of omega-3 fatty acids, you can achieve a much more favorable ratio. This should have long-lasting and often dramatic positive effects on hypertension, heart disease, arthritis, stroke, and other serious maladies.

Because your body cannot manufacture these essential nutrients, they must be obtained from outside sources. Again, cold-water fish and flaxseed are nature's richest sources of the omega-3 fatty acids. Adequate intakes of these bring a much-needed balance between omega-3 EFAs and the more commonly eaten omega-6 EFAs. I recommend eating three to four ounces of cold-water fish such as salmon, herring, or mackerel two or three times a week, or consuming one or two tablespoons of fresh, unprocessed, unheated flaxseed oil daily. (It makes a great salad dressing.) You may also grind ¼ cup raw flaxseed and have it mixed in a drink or sprinkle it on a salad or cereal. However, the easiest way to make sure you're getting enough omega-3 fatty acids is to supplement with fish oil capsules, at least 1,000 milligrams twice a day. For patients who also have high triglycerides and cholesterol, I often increase this to five and occasionally up to ten 1,000-milligram capsules spread out during the day.

COENZYME Q10 FOR HYPERTENSION

Every cell in your body contains coenzyme Q10 (CoQ10), also known as ubiquinone. It is involved in the manufacture of energy in the mitochondria, the powerhouses of the cells. Since your heart is your most metabolically active organ, CoQ10 is naturally more concentrated in this organ. Your body produces its own CoQ10, yet deficiencies are common, especially in patients with hypertension and other cardiovascular diseases. Low levels have been noted in 39 percent of patients with high blood pressure, and heart biopsies of cardiac patients show deficiencies of up to 75 percent when compared with CoQ10 levels in normal heart tissue. Not surprisingly, supplemental coenzyme Q10 has astounding effects on the heart.

One of my patients, 24-year-old Bill, was admitted to the hospital with severe cardiomyopathy, or degeneration of the heart muscle. His lungs were filled with fluid and his heart rhythm was completely erratic. His ejection fraction (an indication of the heart's pumping capacity) was only 17 percent (normal is above 50 percent). Bill's prognosis was dismal—only half of the patients in his condition survive one year. On my recommendation (not that of his cardiologist, who wasn't even familiar with this nondrug therapy), Bill started taking large amounts of CoQ10, as well as other nutritional supplements. Much to his doctor's surprise, he fully recovered. He was able to finish college and is now leading a normal, productive life. He has no activity restrictions, nor is he taking any medications.

The medical literature is full of studies documenting similar "miraculous" recoveries in patients with cardiomyopathy and congestive heart failure after taking CoQ10. A number of important studies confirm the value of CoQ10 in controlling hypertension as well. In a 1994 study conducted at the University of Texas, Dr. Peter Langsjoen and colleagues treated 109 hypertensive patients with an average dose of 225 milligrams of CoQ10 daily, in addition to their prescribed drug regimen. Within five months, a remarkable 51 percent of the patients were able to come off from one to three antihypertensive drugs. In addition, 9.4 percent of the patients were found to have "highly significant" improvements in their diastolic function and the integrity of the left ventricular wall of the heart, the area most affected by hypertension.

Most physicians are still in the dark about CoQ10, even with sufficient evidence showing that low tissue levels of this coenzyme are linked to cardiovascular disease. CoQ10 has tremendous clinical value in the treatment of hypertension, congestive heart failure, cardiomyopathy, and mitral valve prolapse. I have seen excellent results with this supplement and absolutely require my hypertensive patients to take it, in a dose of 180 to 200 milligrams per day. CoQ10 must be taken with fat for proper absorption. Take it with a meal that contains a little healthy fat, or purchase oil-based CoQ10 gelcaps or chewable CoQ10 wafers that contain a small amount of fat. Be patient—it may take four to twelve weeks before the effects of CoQ10 are noticed.

ARGININE: AN AMINO ACID FOR THE HEART

Nitric oxide is currently the subject of intense scientific scrutiny, as this minuscule, short-lived gas molecule has been discovered to play important roles in immunity, aging, male sexual function, cardiovascular health, and the regulation of blood pressure. As I explained in Chapter 2, nitric oxide is released by the endothelial cells lining the arteries and arterioles. It is a potent vasodilator—it relaxes the smooth muscle cells of the arteries, increasing their diameter and lowering blood pressure.

It is also intimately involved in the prevention of atherosclerosis. Atherosclerosis, to review what we discussed in previous chapters, begins with an injury to the endothelial cells. Platelets, white blood cells, and oxidized LDL cholesterol are drawn to the site of the injury, where they take up residence—and it's off to the races for atherosclerosis. As the process continues, your arteries eventually become stiff, narrow, and unresponsive. It has long been thought that the initial damage was due to physical causes—the trauma of high blood pressure or damage caused by an infectious or toxic agent. However, a new theory has emerged in the past few years, and that is that the initial injury to the artery wall may also be caused by impairment in the activity of nitric oxide. In addition to relaxing your blood vessels, nitric oxide also prevents platelets and white blood cells from attaching to arterial walls.

In order for your body to make nitric oxide, it must have adequate supplies of the amino acid arginine. Yet many people don't get enough of this raw material to overcome the factors working against nitric oxide synthesis, such as oxidized LDL cholesterol, which blocks its production. Early research with arginine involved intravenous administration of the amino acid, and it was quite effective in the lowering of blood pressure and the prevention of heart disease. However, more recent studies utilizing oral supplements have demonstrated that oral arginine is also beneficial in the treatment of atherosclerosis and hypertension.

In a 1997 study presented at the American Heart Association's Seventieth Scientific Session, patients with mild to moderate hypertension taking 2 grams of arginine in oral supplement form experienced significant reductions in blood pressure. Another study, conducted in Italy with patients with newly diagnosed borderline hypertension, demonstrated that 2 grams of oral arginine lowered systolic blood pressure by 20 mm Hg after only a week of supplementation!

You get some arginine in your diet, especially if you eat a lot of animal protein. The average American gets a little over 5 grams of this amino acid per day from their diet. The recommended supplemental dose is 1 gram three times a day, although some people require double that dose (2 grams three times a day) to notice benefits. Arginine is sold in 500-milligram capsules or in powders that can be mixed in water. It is quite safe, although a small percentage of people report stomach upset when taking it on an empty stomach. It is therefore recommended that arginine be taken with some carbohydrate-containing food. Avoid eating protein at the same time you are taking arginine, as this may result in less than optimal absorption.

HERBS THAT LOWER BLOOD PRESSURE

Science is finally beginning to recognize what traditional healers have known for centuries: herbs are powerful natural medicines. Many botanical agents have been utilized successfully for the treatment of hypertension for hundreds, perhaps thousands of years. Some, like garlic, can be found right in your own kitchen cupboard. Others, namely hawthorn, may be new to you but are actually time-tested, well-known remedies in other countries.

Garlic

The Latin name for garlic is *Allium sativum*, which comes from the word meaning "all." It's an apt name when you consider garlic's all-encompassing health benefits. Studies show that garlic can reduce blood pressure, lower cholesterol, improve immune function, and help reverse insulin resistance. It is also a heavy metal chelator, meaning it binds to and facilitates the removal of heavy metals, such as lead and mercury, from the bloodstream. Garlic also has the ability to stimulate the production of the amino acid glutathione, a powerful antioxidant and detoxifier. Its sulfur compounds, the best known of which is allicin, appear to be responsible for much of garlic's health-enhancing properties. Another of garlic's natural components, adenosine, is a smooth muscle relaxant that has been shown to effectively reduce high blood pressure.

The Russians have long known about garlic's cardiovascular benefits, and it is reported that they regularly consume garlic-spiked vodka to bring blood pressure down. While the vodka dilates blood vessels and temporarily improves circulation, the garlic reduces blood pressure, cholesterol, and triglycerides. Vodka aside, there is impressive evidence that garlic is a natural antihypertensive. In a 1990 randomized, placebo-controlled, double-blind trial conducted in West Germany, patients with hypertension were divided into two groups and given either a garlic powder preparation or a placebo. After twelve weeks, patients in the garlic group reduced their mean diastolic pressure from an average of 102 to 89 mm Hg, while the placebo group showed no major changes in blood pressure. Serum cholesterol and triglyceride levels were also reduced in the garlic group. Although in other studies the declines in blood pressure have been more modest, they've still been in the respectable range of 8 to 11 mm/Hg systolic and 5 to 8 mm/Hg diastolic range.

How fast can garlic work? This was evaluated in a study of hypertensive rats given an oral garlic extract. The animals' blood pressure was measured immediately before the extract was given and again at regular intervals over a forty-eight-hour period afterward. The researchers found a marked decrease in the systolic blood pressure of all of the rats in as little as thirty minutes. In fact, the reduction was sufficient to return blood pressure to a normal level and sustain it for up to twenty-four hours.

Garlic also benefits those suffering from insulin resistance. It has been shown to decrease circulating blood glucose and improve insulin sensitivity, making it an important supplement for individuals with insulin resistance and any of the components of syndrome X (hypertension, abdominal obesity, elevated blood lipids, and glucose intolerance). Garlic appears to work by stimulating blocked insulin receptors, which researchers suspect has to do with its antioxidant properties.

I recommend that you get as much garlic in your diet as you can. You'll find garlic in several forms—fresh cloves, juice, oil, dehydrated granules, powder, and puree. Garlic salt is the only form I want you to avoid, and for obvious reasons. I've always maintained that fresh is best—one or two cloves per day. However, if you find the taste of garlic unappealing, use supplements. Look for a product that mentions its equivalent of fresh garlic, and take an amount comparable to one to two cloves of garlic per day.

Hawthorn

Hawthorn is a spiny shrub from Europe also known as *Crataegus oxyacantha* (*kratos,* meaning "sharp," and *akantha,* meaning "thorn"). Hawthorn leaves, berries, and blossoms contain many biologically active compounds and are particularly rich in vitexin flavonoids. These unique compounds are responsible for many of the herb's cardiovascular benefits, including increased blood supply to the heart, improved metabolic processes in the heart, the prevention of atherosclerosis, and the reduction of blood pressure. European physicians routinely prescribe hawthorn extracts for heart disease and circulatory problems such as hypertension, congestive heart failure, and angina. Clinical trials also show that hawthorn can lower serum cholesterol levels and prevent arterial plaque buildup.

A powerful natural antihypertensive, hawthorn works in two ways to bring down blood pressure. First, it naturally dilates blood vessels, increasing the diameter of the "pipes" to lower pressure. Hawthorn also inhibits angiotensin-converting enzyme, the same mechanism by which ACE inhibitor drugs work. The difference is that hawthorn has no harmful side effects and instead nourishes and strengthens the entire cardiovascular system. It does, however, take a little longer to work—up to six weeks—so be patient when you try this natural therapy against hypertension. The suggested dose is 360 milligrams daily of a hawthorn extract standardized to contain 1.8 to 2.2 percent vitexin flavonoids.

PUTTING TOGETHER A NUTRITIONAL SUPPLEMENT PROGRAM

We've covered a lot of nutritional supplements in this chapter. With so many important nutrients proven to help reduce blood pressure, you're probably wondering where to begin. Your best bet is to start taking a broad-based, high-quality multiple vitamin and mineral formula. The supplement should contain adequate dosages of the antioxidants and B vitamins discussed in this chapter, along with the blood-pressure-reducing minerals potassium, magnesium, and calcium, and the trace minerals chromium, selenium, zinc, and vanadium (vanadyl sulfate), as discussed in Chapter 9.

A word of warning before you start shopping for a multivitamin and mineral supplement. The ordinary one-a-day type will not begin to contain the nutrient doses recommended in this book. As I stated earlier, the RDAs are ridiculously low, yet they are the standard to which many supplement manufacturers adhere. (See Appendix E for information on where to find high-quality, high-potency nutritional supplements.) If the formulation you choose does not contain all of the nutrients at the potencies you want and need, simply augment them with appropriate doses of single-nutrient supplements. Garlic, hawthorn herbs, vanadyl sulfate, coenzyme Q10, and arginine—and perhaps other nutrients as well, depending on the formula you choose—will need to be purchased separately.

Nutritional supplements are best taken with meals for several reasons. First, fat-soluble nutrients such as coenzyme Q10 and vitamin A need a little dietary fat in order to be properly assimilated. Second, some people experience gastrointestinal discomfort when taking supplements on an empty stomach. And third, it's easier to remember to take your supplements if you always do so with meals. In addition, you should spread them out over the day—at least twice a day. Your body can only use so much of the water-soluble nutrients at any given time. What you can't use will be excreted in your urine. My patients have found that the easiest schedule to maintain is to take supplements with breakfast and again with dinner.

RECOMMENDED NUTRIENTS FOR HYPERTENSION

Nutrient	Recommended Daily Dose
Vitamin A	5,000 international units
Vitamin A (beta-carotene)	15,000 international units
Vitamin C	2,500 milligrams
Vitamin E	800 international units
Vitamin B-6	75 milligrams
Vitamin B-12	100 micrograms
Folic acid	800 micrograms
Calcium	1,000 milligrams
Magnesium	1,000 milligrams
Chromium	200 micrograms
Selenium	200 micrograms
Vanadyl sulfate*	45 milligrams
Zinc	30 milligrams
Fish oil capsules (omega-3 EFAs)	2,000 to 5,000 milligrams
Coenzyme Q10	180 to 200 milligrams
Arginine†	1–2 grams three times per day
Garlic	Supplemental equivalent of 1 to 2 cloves

| Hawthorn | 360 milligrams of an extract standardized for 1.8 to 2.2 percent vitexin flavonoids |

*Higher doses of vanadyl sulfate should be taken only under the close monitoring of your physician.

†Start with 1 gram 3 times a day and build up to 2 grams three times a day, if needed. For best absorption avoid eating protein at the same time you take arginine.

CHAPTER 11

The Whitaker Wellness Diet for High Blood Pressure

Twenty-seven-year-old John received the shock of his life when he failed the physical required as part of his application for a job with the county. His blood pressure was 160/110! How could he have hypertension? He was young and had no health problems or family history of cardiovascular disease, yet repeated monitoring indicated that he did indeed have hypertension. John's diagnosis didn't surprise me as much as it did him. In spite of his relatively young age, he had all the characteristics of insulin resistance. Although he had been quite active as a teenager, he had significantly slowed down over the last few years. He admitted that his diet was pretty sorry and that he drank more than his share of beer. He was 35 pounds over his "fighting weight," and he carried it in his belly. Furthermore, he had elevated cholesterol, triglycerides, and uric acid.

John needed to bring down his blood pressure, and he needed to bring it down fast. His mother, who is a family friend, asked for advice, and I recommended she put him on what we call the Quick Start Diet for High Blood Pressure. For two weeks, he was to eat all the vegetables, fruit, and rice he wanted—but nothing else. This is not the normal diet I recommend for patients with hypertension, but it has been demonstrated time and again to bring blood pressure down in a hurry. Two weeks later, John's blood pressure was rechecked, and it was a normal 130/60. He was switched to the more liberal Whitaker Wellness Diet, and after another two weeks he had lost a total of 13 pounds, his cholesterol had fallen from 231 to 168, his triglycerides hovered just above normal, and his blood pressure remained in the normal range. John got the job—but more important, he got a wakeup call about his health and saved himself from serious complications down the road.

Imagine yourself at the Whitaker Wellness Institute, sitting down to a meal prepared by Idel Kelly, the chef who has been working with me and preparing meals for my patients for almost twenty years. You are seated at a table with other patients, perhaps discussing the lectures you heard earlier in the day and engaging in pleasant dinner conversation. The first course you are served is a salad of fresh greens, garnished with tomato and cucumber and dressed with a light olive oil, lemon, and garlic dressing. Next on the menu is the main course; tonight it's broiled salmon with yogurt-dill sauce on the side, couscous, and several pencil-thin asparagus spears. Dessert is a poached pear with vanilla yogurt sauce, served with a cup of herbal tea or decaffeinated coffee. Could you get used to this?

Only the most dedicated meat-and-potato eaters complain of the food served during the weeklong program at the Institute. For most, the soups and salads, the quiches and tostadas, the fish and chicken, are completely satisfying, tasty, and filling. No, you can't borrow Idel—she's much too valuable to me. But I will share with you in this chapter the basics of the food program we employ at the clinic for reversing hypertension. And in Appendix C I'll provide two weeks of menu plans and recipes to help you get started.

Dietary changes are among the most effective and attractive parts of this program for reversing hypertension. You will discover that the food choices and recipes recommended for lowering blood pressure are varied, delicious, and easy to prepare. You'll be pleasantly surprised at how rapidly your blood pressure will respond to these dietary modifications, particularly when used in conjunction with the other therapies recommended in this book. And because this diet addresses the nutrient imbalances and insulin resistance that underlie hypertension and other maladies, it will improve many facets of your health. It will likely help you lose weight and give you more energy, lower your cholesterol and triglyceride levels, and normalize your blood pressure. It may even improve other, seemingly unrelated medical conditions that have bothered you for years.

THE DASH STUDY: DIETARY APPROACHES TO STOP HYPERTENSION

One of the most ambitious research efforts ever mounted to explore the effects of a therapeutic diet on blood pressure was the Dietary Approaches to Stop Hypertension (DASH) Trial published in 1997. This randomized controlled clinical study, which was carried out at four university medical centers, involved 459 adults with untreated high normal blood pressure to mild hypertension (systolic less than 160 mm Hg and diastolic 85 to 90 mm Hg). These patients, whose age averaged 44.6 years, were divided into three groups: 1) a control group, in which participants consumed a typical high-fat American diet; 2) a group who ate a typical high-fat American diet but increased their intake of fruits and vegetables; 3) a group whose diet included fruits, vegetables, low-fat dairy products, and foods reduced in saturated fat (called the "combination" diet because it combined the characteristics researchers presumed would lower blood pressure). All the groups were fed the control diet for three weeks before starting on their assigned diets.

After eight weeks patients on the DASH combination diet experienced an average lowering of blood pressure of 11.4 mm Hg systolic and 5.5 mm Hg diastolic. When researchers compared the effects of this diet with the effects of drug therapy using one antihypertensive medication, they concluded that the combination diet could serve as an alternative to drug therapy for patients with stage 1 (mild) hypertension. The blood-pressure-lowering effects of this diet were predicted to reduce the incidence of coronary heart disease by 15 percent and the incidence of stroke by 27 percent, nationwide. All this from low-tech, unsexy changes in diet!

The findings of the DASH study didn't surprise me one bit. For twenty-five years I have observed in my patients that a diet low in total and saturated fats and rich in fruits and vegetables can significantly reduce blood pressure. But what I find so thrilling about this large-scale study is that it finally proves that *diet alone can reduce blood pressure as effectively as antihypertensive drug therapy*—without the side effects of drugs!

THE HEALTH BENEFITS OF A PLANT-BASED DIET

The DASH combination diet is quite similar to the diet that I recommend for the treatment and prevention of hypertension and many other medical conditions. While my diet does include fish, skinless poultry, and low-fat dairy products, its central focus is on fresh fruits and vegetables, whole grains, and legumes. These foods are naturally very low in sodium and contain lots of potassium, ensuring that your potassium-sodium ratio is at its optimum (four parts potassium to one part sodium—the K Factor discussed in Chapter 8). They are also low in saturated fat and provide the essential antioxidants, vitamins, and minerals discussed in Chapters 9 and 10. The greater emphasis on plant foods is the primary difference between the Whitaker Wellness Diet and the DASH combination diet.

In addition to antioxidants, vitamins, and minerals, fruits and vegetables provide a vast array of phytochemicals, specialized compounds in plants that protect them from the harsh realities of their environments—and confer health benefits when eaten. Scores of phytochemicals have been identified in recent years, and research into their effects on human health is in full swing. One important class of phytochemicals is flavonoids, which give plants their colors and possess powerful antioxidant activity. Flavonoids in fruits and vegetables strengthen your blood vessels and connective tissue, and their effects are even stronger when they are taken with vitamin C.

▼ SENSATIONAL CELERY

Celery for hypertension? Before you scoff, read this. Celery contains a compound called 3-n-butyl-phthalide, which has been demonstrated in animal studies to lower blood pressure by 12 to 14 percent. Researchers at the University of

Chicago Medical Center decided to look into celery's effects on blood pressure when the father of one of the scientists noted a drop in his blood pressure from 158/96 to 118/82 after eating ¼ pound of celery daily for one week. The amount of 3-n-butyl-phthalide used in the animal study equates to that found in four stalks of celery.

Dietary flavonoids also offer protection against stroke. In a 1996 study published in the *Archives of Internal Medicine*, 552 men aged 50 to 69 years were followed for fifteen years, during which time their average nutrient and food intake was periodically evaluated through detailed dietary histories. The researchers found that there was indeed a direct connection between the amount of flavonoids consumed and the incidence of stroke. When flavonoid intake was high (especially quercetin, which is most concentrated in yellow onions), stroke incidence was significantly reduced. Other studies have shown that a high flavonoid intake correlates with a low risk of heart attack and heart disease.

I recommend that you eat plenty of onions, citrus fruits, and berries—excellent sources of flavonoids. Green tea and red wine are also rich in these beneficial phytochemicals and may be consumed in moderation. The point, however, is not to concentrate only on flavonoids but to reap the benefits of many phytochemicals by incorporating a variety of fruits and vegetables into your diet.

▼ PHYTOCHEMICALS AND THEIR BENEFITS

Here is a list of some of the best-studied phytochemicals, their sources, and their benefits for your health.

Phytochemical	Food Source	Benefits
Carotenoids	Leafy greens	Powerful antioxidant activity
Allicin	Garlic	Lowers blood pressure and cholesterol, enhances immune activity

Bioflavonoids and liminoid	Citrus fruits	Reduce tumor growth and promote production of detoxifying enzymes
Ellagic acid	Strawberries and cherries	Antioxidant activity
Lutein and zeaxanthin	Leafy greens	Protect eyes from ultraviolet damage

Epidemiological research, which involves the study of distinct populations to determine the relationships between environmental factors and disease, supports the benefits of a primarily plant-based diet. Among traditional hunter-gatherer societies, such as the natives of New Guinea and the Carajas Indians of Brazil, who subsist on vegetables, fruits, and some wild game, hypertension, as well as stroke and heart attacks, are almost nonexistent. Vegetarians in industrialized countries likewise have a low incidence of hypertension and heart disease. A 1977 study published in the *American Journal of Epidemiology* compared the vegetarian diet of Seventh-Day Adventists with that of meat eaters and found a significantly lower incidence of heart disease among the vegetarians. Other studies of vegetarians have noted similar trends, suggesting that plant foods protect against hypertension.

The Whitaker Wellness Diet takes this epidemiological evidence and combines it with the newest scientific discoveries regarding hypertension. Before we get into the details, however, I'd like to introduce those of you with severely elevated blood pressure to my Quick Start Diet for High Blood Pressure, described on pages 144–46. The purpose of this diet is to bring your blood pressure down quickly and safely. If your blood pressure is dangerously high—stage 3: systolic over 180 mm Hg or diastolic over 110 mm Hg—try this diet for one to six weeks, under your doctor's supervision, until your blood pressure falls to more normal levels. Then continue with the Whitaker Wellness Diet for High Blood Pressure described later in this chapter.

▽ | THE QUICK START DIET FOR HIGH BLOOD PRESSURE

For some folks, hypertension is not only a health risk but also a job risk. Commercial pilots, for instance, are routinely checked for hypertension and are not allowed to use medication to bring down high blood pressure. Their solution? A healthy diet. One of my patients is an airline pilot in his early fifties, and he almost lost his pilot's license because of hypertension. He had less than three weeks to bring it down without medication, so I put him on the Quick Start Diet. To his amazement, his blood pressure plummeted from a dangerous 225/115 to a healthy 130/84 in just twelve days! A week later he passed his flight physical exam with "flying colors" and is still flying to this day. John, the 27-year-old I told you about in the opening of this chapter, had a similar experience.

The Quick Start Diet these patients followed is very simple: rice, fruit, and vegetables. That's it. It was originally designed in the 1940s by Dr. Walter Kempner, of Duke University, who called it the rice-fruit diet (even though it included vegetables). This diet is naturally low in salt, fat, and protein and extremely high in dietary potassium, magnesium, antioxidants, complex carbohydrates, fiber, and other important nutrients. Dr. Kempner was able to demonstrate that these dietary changes could return high blood pressure to normal. In most cases, he was able to reduce blood pressure in hypertensives by at least 20 mm Hg—with no other interventions. With results of this magnitude, you'd expect the medical community to stand up and take notice. However, as with other nutritional therapies, the effectiveness of Dr. Kempner's diet was ignored by the medical establishment.

Let's not wait for conventional medicine to catch up with what we already know. The Quick Start Diet works. So if your blood pressure has been classified as stage 3, I would suggest that, under your doctor's supervision, for one to six weeks you eat steamed brown rice, fresh fruit, and vegetables to your heart's delight—but nothing else. You may steam, broil, roast, poach, or sauté the vegetables (in water, not oil) and season them with lemon or herbs. For a sweetener, use only stevia, a natural herb sweetener that is sold in health food stores. But during this brief period don't use any other grains, legumes, oil, salt-containing spices, corn, alcohol, meat, or dairy products. Consult the recommended foods list at the end of this chapter for suggested fruits and vegetables. You'll be pleased to discover that rice with vegetables and herbal seasonings can make a delicious meal, and fresh fruit is a delightful snack. Eat organic fruits and vegetables if you can find them, and enjoy them fresh whenever possible. Caffeinated beverages are not allowed on the Quick Start Diet; if you must have your coffee in the morning, drink decaffeinated or a coffee substitute. Your fluid intake should be mostly water, and you should drink plenty of it, although herbal teas are fine, too. The Quick Start Diet may seem quite restrictive at first, but isn't your health worth a few weeks of disciplined eating? Here's a sample day's menu.

Breakfast: Blueberries and brown rice (sweetened with stevia)
Snack: Grapefruit
Lunch: Homemade vegetable soup (recipe in Appendix C)
   Green salad with lemon juice and herb dressing
Snack: Apple wedges
Dinner: Brown rice topped with sliced mushrooms sautéed in
   water and Italian herbs
   Steamed broccoli and cauliflower
Dessert: Sliced strawberries

Don't worry about quantities—nobody ever got fat or sick by overeating salad and zucchini. It's hard to eat too much of these foods. Mix up your fruits and vegetables for variety. Use fresh herbs to flavor your rice and vegetables. Don't forget that this is a short-term diet with long-term benefits. Remember, too, that this Quick Start Diet is not for everyone. In fact, for prolonged periods it's not for anyone. But it has been scientifically proven to bring elevated blood pressure down fast. If you have stage 3 hypertension, this therapeutic diet is a must. Here are a few tips to get you off to a good "Quick Start."

- See your doctor before implementing this diet.
- Keep track of your progress by monitoring your blood pressure daily.
- Drink twelve 8-ounce glasses of water per day.
- Take a high-quality multivitamin and mineral supplement daily as described in Chapter 10.

After your blood pressure is back in a more normal range, I would suggest you move on to the Whitaker Wellness Diet for High Blood Pressure.

THE WHITAKER WELLNESS DIET FOR
HIGH BLOOD PRESSURE

Although the Quick Start Diet is ideal for quickly and safely bringing down severely elevated blood pressure, it is too limiting to sustain beyond the one to six weeks I recommend. So I've developed a more moderate, lifelong eating plan for blood pressure reduction and maintenance. Let's look at the guiding principles of the Whitaker Wellness Diet for High Blood Pressure.

Good Fats/Bad Fats

Fat has such a bad reputation that we sometimes forget that it has very important biologic functions in our bodies. Fat can be stored and burned for energy. It is important for the transport of the fat-soluble nutrients, which include vitamins A, D, E, and K. Fat also cushions your organs, insulates your body, helps regulate body temperature, and is an essential structural component of your cell membranes. Certain fats, such as those discussed in Chapter 10, are precursors to prostaglandins, which have a positive impact on blood pressure. It is, however, important to consider the kinds of fat you eat. Some fats are downright dangerous and have no place in a health-promoting diet, others are of vital importance for optimal health.

One type of fat you should avoid is saturated fat, which comes mostly from animal sources. Saturated fat can be identified by one simple characteristic: it is solid at room temperature. Saturated fat contributes to heart disease and high blood pressure because it thickens the blood and is easily deposited in the artery walls. As these deposits accumulate, the arteries narrow and blood pressure is driven up. Saturated animal fats are loaded with cholesterol, another culprit in cardiovascular disease. In fact, dietary cholesterol is *only* found in animal products; it is especially prevalent in red meats, egg yolks, and whole-fat dairy products. These are among the foods I recommend you for the most part avoid.

With this in mind, it would seem that vegetable-derived fats would be a far healthier choice. While it is true that legumes, vegetables, nuts, seeds, and grains in their natural state contain small amounts of wonderful, heart-healthy fats, these fats are very fragile and easily damaged by heat, air, light, or chemicals. Most of the vegetable oils sold in your supermarket have been extracted with harsh chemicals at high temperatures, bleached, and otherwise altered. (Extra-virgin olive oil, because it is so easily extracted, is a healthy exception.) Stay away from these processed vegetable oils. Instead, look in your health food store for *expeller-pressed* vegetable oils. The best ones come in dark bottles that protect them from light, and they should be stored in the refrigerator or freezer to retain their freshness.

One type of processed fats I urge you to avoid is *hydrogenated fats*. Margarine and solid vegetable shortening, which is found in most commercial baked goods, are examples of hydrogenated fats. Hydrogenated fats are polyunsaturated vegetable oils that have been transformed, through a heat and chemical process, into dangerous *trans fatty acids* (TFAs). Hydrogenation makes liquid vegetable oils solid at room temperature and extends their shelf life, which is good for the grocer but not for you. Once they are in your body, trans fatty acids interfere with the basic functions of natural fats. They raise LDL cholesterol and lower HDL cholesterol, increasing your risk of stroke and heart attack. According to Harvard researcher Walter Willet, consumption of these unnatural fats may cause 30,000 deaths a year.

TFAs have also been linked to increased risk of diabetes, infertility, obesity, and immune dysfunction.

On the other hand, there are healthy fats that you should most definitely include in your diet. Raw nuts, seeds, and nut butters make excellent snacks and are a good source of protein and healthy fats. One of the healthiest oils is flaxseed oil, a polyunsaturated fat that contains omega-3 essential fatty acids (EFAs). While it makes a great salad dressing, like all EFAs it is extremely fragile and should not be heated or used for cooking. The most practical oils for cooking are those high in monounsaturated fats, especially olive oil and hazelnut oil. Monounsaturated oils are more stable and less prone to being harmfully altered by processing and cooking than polyunsaturated oils such as sunflower, safflower, corn, and most other vegetable oils. Yet even monounsaturated oils should be handled gingerly (they can only take medium heat—less than 325°) and eaten in prudent quantities.

The quantity and quality of fats consumed definitely affect blood pressure. Consider the research of Dr. P. Pusha, who studied 57 couples living in northern Finland, an area noted for its high heart attack death rate. These couples were separated into three groups to determine what effect dietary changes had on blood pressure. Group one reduced their fat intake from 40 percent of daily calories (similar to the American fat intake) to about 20 percent and ate primarily polyunsaturated vegetable oils. Group two reduced their salt intake by 50 percent (from 10 grams of salt daily to 5 grams). Group three made no changes. The only group that experienced significant lowering of blood pressure was the first group, which lowered fat intake and ate primarily polyunsaturated fats. Their average systolic blood pressure dropped 8.9 mm Hg and their diastolic 6.6 mm Hg. This reduction was not due to weight loss or any factor other than the type and amount of fat they consumed.

I recommend that you obtain about 20 percent of your daily calories from healthy fats, while avoiding animal-source saturated fats and hydrogenated trans fatty acids such as margarine and processed vegetable oils. Buy expeller-pressed polyunsaturated vegetable oils only and store them in your refrigerator. A good rule of thumb is to never heat polyunsaturated vegetable oils, since frying, roasting, or heat processing robs them of their health benefits. Should you occasionally need to use oil for baking or cooking, use monounsaturated oil—extra-virgin olive oil and hazelnut oil are the best. These oils are considerably more stable than polyunsaturated oils.

Federal law mandates that all packaged foods indicate how many grams of fat are included in each serving. Learning to read food labels is a tried and true way to eliminate hidden fat from your diet. To read a label for fat content, first check the total number of calories per serving, as well as the number of calories from fat per serving. Then compute a simple percentage by dividing fat calories by total calories. If, for example, a food has 30 fat calories and 90 total calories, 33 percent of its calories come from fat (30÷90). And remember, if the food contains processed fat (look for "partially hydrogenated" or "hydrogenated" on the label), it should be avoided, regardless of how much fat it contains.

Protein Power

Protein is one of the most important nutrients required by the human body. People often equate protein with muscle, but your muscles aren't the only part of your body made of protein. Approximately half of the solid substances of your body are composed of protein—it is required for the construction of hair, nerves, skin, blood, sperm, and eggs. Protein also provides the basic building blocks for enzymes, hormones, blood plasma, and even saliva. However, most Americans eat more protein than they need. Excess protein is hard on the kidneys and can also contribute to osteoporosis, or thinning of the bones, as we age. Furthermore, high-protein foods such as meat and whole dairy also contain a lot of fat, much of it unhealthy saturated fat.

I recommend that you get about 20 percent of your daily total calories from protein, concentrating on lean protein sources such as fish and seafood, skinless poultry, egg whites (an occasional yolk is fine), low-fat or fat-free dairy products, tofu, legumes, and whole grains. Fish is especially recommended, particularly salmon, herring, mackerel, and other fish rich in omega-3 oils. Increased consumption of such fish is associated with decreases in blood pressure in hypertensive men and women. A plant-based diet, as long as it includes soy

Nutrition Facts

Serving Size 1/2 cup (114g)
Servings Per Container 4

Amount Per Serving

Calories 90   Calories from Fat 30

	% Daily Value*
Total Fat 3g	**5%**
Saturated Fat 0g	**0%**
Cholesterol 0mg	**0%**
Sodium 300mg	**13%**
Total Carbohydrate 13g	**4%**
Dietary Fiber 3g	**12%**
Sugars 3g	
Protein 3g	

Vitamin A	80%	•	Vitamin C	60%
Calcium	4%	•	Iron	4%

* Percent Daily Values are based on a 2,000
calorie diet. Your daily values may be higher or
lower depending on your calorie needs:

	Calories	2,000	2,500
Total Fat	Less than	65g	80g
Sat. Fat	Less than	20g	25g
Cholesterol	Less than	300mg	300mg
Sodium	Less than	2,400mg	2,400mg
Total Carbohydrate		300g	375g
Fiber		25g	30g

Calories per gram:
Fat 9   •   Carbohydrate 4   •   Protein 4

More nutrients may be listed on some labels.

Figure 8. How to Read Food Labels

and other legumes, will provide adequate protein. Aim for three to
four small servings of protein-rich foods per day, and make sure you
eat some protein at each meal.

Carbohydrates: The Right Stuff

Carbohydrates are your body's main source of energy. Through the complex process of digestion, carbohydrates are metabolized into glucose, the fuel that runs everything from the actions inside a single cell to the muscle movements required to lift a weight. Carbohydrates are an important part of a healthy diet. They are the primary component of fruits, vegetables, legumes, and grains. They also make up the bulk of cookies, pretzels, candy, and sodas. It is therefore obvious that not all carbohydrates are equal, and the type of carbohydrates you eat may have a direct bearing on your health—and your blood pressure.

As I explained in Chapter 6, hypertension is often part and parcel of a complex called syndrome X that also includes obesity, high triglycerides and cholesterol, and blood sugar irregularities. The underlying condition in syndrome X is insulin resistance, and for individuals with insulin resistance a very real connection exists between the type of carbohydrates consumed, the release of glucose and insulin, and insulin sensitivity. Choosing foods that release glucose slowly into the bloodstream delays insulin secretion and averts the devastating effects of insulin resistance—including hypertension.

Carbohydrates generally fall into two categories. The *simple sugars* are composed of very basic one- or two-sugar molecules, as found in sucrose (white sugar), brown sugar, molasses, honey, corn syrup, maple syrup, maltose, dextrose, fructose (fruit sugar), and lactose (milk sugar). In fact, any food ending in "-ose" is classified as a simple sugar. Shortly after being eaten, most simple sugars are quickly and easily broken down into glucose, which is then released into the bloodstream. The sudden escalation in blood glucose is followed by an immediate rise in serum insulin.

The second category—*complex carbohydrates*—is found in vegetables, legumes, and whole grains. Complex carbohydrates consist of multiple sugar molecules that are bonded together. Since enzymes are required to break these bonds before they can be transformed into glucose for energy, complex carbohydrates generally take longer to bring about a rise in blood insulin. Complex carbohydrates also contain *fiber*, the indigestible roughage and pectin in unprocessed plant foods. Fiber further slows down the process of insulin release. The whole foods I recommend in the Whitaker Wellness Diet are high in complex carbohydrates and fiber, which allows for a slower release of glucose and insulin into the bloodstream. These are the foods nature designed us to eat for good health.

Unfortunately, there has been a shift in this country toward a diet high in sugar and processed, or refined, carbohydrates. We've taken a healthy grain such as whole wheat and ground it, bleached it, stripped it of its fiber, and robbed it of its nutrients. The result is a concentrated source of empty carbohydrate calories. These highly processed foods are convenient, tasty, and offer a quick boost of energy because they are rapidly converted into glucose. Today's popular low-fat diet fads have exacerbated the problem. In an effort to avoid fat, many people are turning to low-fat foods loaded with refined carbohydrates. Over the past few years, we've seen the introduction of dozens of new categories of these schizophrenic foods—low-fat or nonfat cookies, crackers, chips, ice cream, and cakes. But check the labels on some of these foods the next time you're in the grocery store and you'll see that, although they may contain little or no fat, most are basically a mixture of refined flour and sugar in one of its many guises. These foods aren't good for any of us, but they are particularly detrimental to individuals with syndrome X, the unwelcome complex of metabolic disorders caused by insulin resistance.

GLYCEMIC GUIDELINES

More recent research has added another variable to food evaluation. It's called the *glycemic index*. This is a set of values assigned to foods that describes the rate at which blood glucose rises two or three hours after they are eaten. The standard for the glycemic index is glucose or white bread, each of which metabolizes quite quickly. All other foods are compared to this standard, and the higher the glycemic index value of a food, the quicker and greater the blood glucose response. High glycemic index foods cause sudden, unstable swings in glucose and insulin levels, which in turn contribute to insulin resistance, obesity, hypertension, and glucose intolerance. Foods with a low glycemic index, on the other hand, promote a slower, more sustained release of glucose and insulin. These foods stick with you longer, minimizing hunger, and do not contribute to insulin resistance.

Now, it might seem that all simple sugars would have a high glycemic index value, while all complex carbohydrates (especially those high in fiber) would be low on the glycemic index. But some startling aspects of this research show that certain complex carbohydrate foods—primarily high-starch foods such as potatoes and breads—are in the high-glycemic category. This means they cause a rapid rise of blood glucose and insulin, similar to the body's response to a simple sugar. Also surprising is the fact that some foods that contain simple sugars, such as fruit, have a lower glycemic index, meaning they prompt blood sugar to rise gradually.

Take a look at the list of high glycemic index foods. Some of them are foods you've always been told are healthy for you. Well, they may be healthy for some people, but if your high blood pressure is accompanied by insulin resistance, as it is for so many, it's best to minimize your consumption of these foods.

▼ "HEALTH FOODS" WITH A HIGH GLYCEMIC INDEX VALUE

These foods are not good choices for insulin resistance and hypertension. The list of recommended foods later in this chapter will put you on the right track in making good food choices.

- Most breads
- Crackers and rice cakes
- Corn
- White potatoes
- Tropical fruits
- Most cold cereals

Regardless of the type of carbohydrate you consume, it is eventually broken down into glucose. Your body will use enough glucose to meet your immediate energy needs and what isn't used for energy will be converted into glycogen and stored in the muscles or liver until your energy requirements trigger its conversion back to glucose. Your muscles and liver can hold only so much glycogen; once they are filled to capacity, any glucose left over is converted to and stored as fat. Aside from the obvious ensuing weight gain, overeating of carbohydrates—especially the "quick-release" variety—also causes an increase in triglycerides and cholesterol, which is part and parcel of syndrome X.

Once glucose is utilized for energy or stored, blood glucose levels begin to fall. Because high glycemic index carbohydrates are converted so quickly, their rapid release of glucose—accompanied by elevated insulin levels and a quick energy spurt—is followed by a precipitous drop in blood glucose. This is why patients with insulin resistance often feel tired and hungry: they have either too much glucose in their bloodstream or not enough. Low glycemic index foods (which includes most vegetables, legumes, and fruits), on the other hand, promote a slow, sustained delivery of glucose and insulin. There are no instant highs or dramatic lows, so your blood glucose levels are more stable, and you feel more energetic and satiated throughout the day.

Although fat and protein do not in and of themselves raise glucose levels, they do affect glucose utilization and insulin resistance. Studies show that a high-fat diet reduces cells' sensitivity to insulin, increases triglycerides, and contributes to obesity. At the same time, research shows that, when consumed in prudent amounts, polyunsaturated vegetable oils and cold-water fish oils can improve insulin sensitivity. On the other hand protein, although it elicits an insulin response, stimulates the production of a hormone that helps mobilize the body's fat stores. Therefore, I recommend that all meals contain a little protein and that you take care to cut back on excess fat, while incorporating into your diet the healthy fats discussed earlier in this chapter.

LET DIET MAKE A DIFFERENCE IN YOUR LIFE

If you have high blood pressure, I urge you to try the Whitaker Wellness Diet for High Blood Pressure for at least one month. During this month I want you to eat lots of vegetables, fruits, legumes and whole grains, and moderate amounts of lean protein, while avoiding fatty, salty, processed foods and refined sugars and carbohydrates. Give it a try and see how much of a difference it makes in your life. Let me assure you, you won't go hungry. This is not bland, spartan fare. Nor is it strictly vegetarian, although if you choose to go that route, you can simply replace the chicken or fish with equal amounts of tofu, beans, or a soy-based meat substitute.

After reviewing the categories below and familiarizing yourself with the recommended foods, sample menus, and recipes in Appendix C, you should have everything you need to start on your new diet for reversing hypertension.

Protein Foods

Eat plenty of tofu, beans, egg whites (an occasional yolk is fine), fish, lean chicken, and lean turkey. Avoid pork, veal, and beef. Also, make sure all meat products are free of nitrates, nitrites, sugars, starches, and preservatives. Meat should be prepared in a healthy way—broiled, baked, or grilled. Fry or sauté in water, wine, or broth, not fat. Use only eggs or fresh, frozen, or refrigerated egg-white products. Nonfat yogurt, buttermilk, and skim milk are also permitted. Acceptable cheeses include low-fat or fat-free cottage cheese, farmer's cheese, ricotta, mozzarella, and higher-fat cheeses in moderation. For reasons other than blood pressure control, I don't recommend going overboard on dairy—most people don't tolerate it well. I suggest three or four servings of protein foods every day—approximately 20 percent of your daily caloric intake. A single serving of meat or another animal protein is four to six ounces, about the size of a deck of cards. For other foods, a single serving consists of one-half cup cooked beans, four tablespoons nuts and seeds, two tablespoons nut butter, four to six ounces of tofu, one cup nonfat or low-fat yogurt or cottage cheese, or one cup soy milk.

▼ WHITAKER WELLNESS DIET FOR HIGH BLOOD PRESSURE IN A NUTSHELL

Food	Servings per day	Sample Serving
Protein Foods	3–4	4–6 ounces meat or tofu
		½ cup cooked beans
		4 tablespoons raw nuts and seeds
		4 egg whites
		2 tablespoons nut butter
		1 cup low-fat or nonfat yogurt, cottage cheese, or soy milk
		1–2 ounces low-fat cheese
Grains and Breads	3–4	1 cup cooked whole grains
		1 cup whole-grain cereal
		1 cup cooked pasta
		1 slice bread
Fruits and Vegetables	3–4 servings fruit	1 medium whole fruit
		½ cup sliced fruit
	5–8 servings vegetables	1 cup raw vegetables
		½ cup cooked vegetables

Grains and Breads

Good grains include barley, bulgur, and kasha. Buckwheat and soy flour are excellent choices for baking and making pancakes or waffles. Experiment with flours made from any of the above grains in your favorite recipes. Pasta is okay, but remember to cook it al dente (still somewhat firm), to keep the glycemic index rating low. The longer you cook pasta—or rice, for that matter—the higher the glycemic value. Otherwise, avoid all wheat flour (whole wheat and white), refined starches, breads, bagels, cookies, and crackers. Breads and bagels made with sprouted wheat and other grains, however, are acceptable, as is 100 percent whole rye bread. Limit grain foods to three or four servings per day. One serving equals one cup of cooked whole grains, whole-grain cereals or pasta, or one slice of bread.

Fruits and Vegetables

Most fruits and vegetables are great. Exceptions are those with a high glycemic index value, such as corn, many root vegetables, and tropical fruits, which should be eaten in moderation. Vegetables should be the focus of your meals, and I recommend eating five to eight servings every day. (One serving is one cup raw or one-half cup cooked vegetables.) Limit high-glycemic vegetables such as corn and white potatoes to twice a week each. Also eat three or four servings of fruit (one medium whole fruit or one-half cup sliced fruit) daily.

Fats

Limit added fat to one to two tablespoons of oil per day. Flaxseed and olive oil is best, and it makes a great salad dressing. (Use your favorite recipe but substitute flaxseed or olive oil, or try the recipe on pages 239–40.) Other unprocessed polyunsaturated oils, provided that they are expeller-pressed and kept refrigerated, are okay in small amounts. Never heat these oils; for cooking, your best bets are olive oil and hazelnut oil. Avoid saturated fats and trans fatty acids, including margarine, cream, and regular mayonnaise. (Like the Italians, dip your bread in a small amount of virgin olive oil rather than using butter or margarine.) Remember, you'll be getting small amounts of fat in beans, grains, nuts and seeds, and lean animal protein foods.

Seasonings

I encourage you to start using fresh or dried herbs to flavor your foods. Garlic is an especially tasty and healthy seasoning. Add it to salads, pastas, and soups. You can counteract bad breath by chewing fresh parsley, mint, or citrus peel, and rid your hands of odor by rubbing them over your kitchen faucet. (This sounds strange, but it works.) Experiment with the delightful tastes of basil in your salad dressing, parsley or dill with your fish dishes, and oregano, rosemary, or thyme with chicken. These herbs can truly transform an ordinary meal into a gourmet event. For a salty taste without the danger of sodium chloride, you could try a potassium salt such as Nu-Salt or NoSalt, or you could use the sea vegetable dulse. (For a detailed discussion of sodium, refer to Chapter 8.)

Sweeteners

Sucrose (white sugar), brown sugar, and even honey are very high on the glycemic index. More acceptable sugars—used in moderation—include xylitol and brown rice syrup. The best of all sweeteners is stevia, a natural, noncaloric, herb-based sweetener available in health food stores. It can be used to flavor hot cereals, beverages, and baked goods. Also try sweet spices such as cinnamon and nutmeg. Avoid artificial sweeteners, particularly aspartame (Nutrasweet).

Beverages

I recommend drinking ten to twelve eight-ounce glasses of water per day. (See Chapter 12 for more on how water affects blood pressure.) Clean, purified water is best. For variety try sodium-free seltzer water, flavored with lemon or lime. Iced herbal teas are also good. No alcohol is allowed on the Quick Start Diet; one to two drinks per day are acceptable on the Whitaker Wellness Diet. Avoid sodas and any artificially sweetened beverages. Fruit juices contain way too much concentrated sugar and should be drunk in moderation—and diluted with water, at that. Caffeine tends to raise blood pressure in some people, so it should be avoided. Decaffeinated coffee and tea are acceptable. If you feel you need an occasional jolt of caffeine, have a cup of green tea, which has less caffeine than coffee and also contains many beneficial phytochemicals.

▼ RECOMMENDED FOODS FOR THE WHITAKER WELLNESS DIET FOR HIGH BLOOD PRESSURE

Here is a detailed list of recommended foods for the Whitaker Wellness Diet for High Blood Pressure. These foods all have relatively low glycemic index values as determined by the Glycemic Research Institute in Washington, D.C. (See Appendix E for more information.)

Fruits (Fresh and Frozen)

Apple

Applesauce (unsweetened)

Bananas (Although the glycemic index of bananas is high, they
    contain lots of potassium, as well as other compounds that
    may lower blood pressure.) Bananas have a much lower
    glycemic response if they are not too ripe. They should have
    some green on the skin. Limit to no more than one a day.

Blackberries

Blueberries

Boysenberries

Cantaloupe

Cherries

Figs

Grapefruit

Grapes (limit to 5–10 grapes)

Honeydew melons

Lemon

Lime

Mandarin orange

Nectarine

Orange

Peach

Pear

Persimmon

Plum

Pomegranate

Raspberries
Strawberries
Tangerine

Canned Fruit

Peaches in their own juice
Pears in their own juice

Jams and Jellies (Use in Moderation)

Jams and jellies, without corn syrup or added sucrose. Limit to
one tablespoon.

Vegetables

Artichoke
Arugula
Asparagus
Avocado
Bean sprouts
Bell pepper
Broccoli
Brussels sprouts
Cabbage
Cauliflower
Celery
Collard greens
Eggplant
Endive
Escarole
Green beans
Green pepper
Kale
Kohlrabi
Leeks
Lettuce
Mushrooms
Mustard greens
Okra

Olives

Onions

Pea pods

Peppers (hot)

Radishes

Red pepper

Rutabaga

Sauerkraut

Scallions

Snow peas

Spinach

Squash (summer yellow)

Sweet potatoes (not yams)

Tomatoes

Turnip greens

Water chestnuts

Zucchini

Legumes

Cook beans without salt. Dried, fresh, and frozen beans have a lower glycemic index than canned. If you use canned beans, rinse them well in a colander to remove much of the salt.

Black beans

Black-eyed peas

Butter beans

Garbanzo beans (chickpeas)

Kidney beans

Lentils, green or regular

Lima beans

Navy beans

Peas, green

Soybeans

White haricot

Breads

Most breads are very high on the glycemic index. Here are a few exceptions.

100% sprouted-wheat bread, pita, bagels, etc.
100% stone-ground whole wheat crackers
100% whole-grain rye bread
Pumpernickel made with 100% rye
Whole wheat pita
Whole wheat tortillas

Cereals

Buckwheat kasha
Oat groats
Oatmeal (long-cooking, not quick-cooking)
Pearled barley cereal
Quinoa
Teff
Wheat bran

Pasta

Almost all pastas are acceptable. (Canned pastas and gnocchi made from potatoes are not.) Boil pasta just until it is cooked al dente, since this keeps its glycemic response in the lower range.

Pasta Sauces

Use sauces made without corn syrup or sugar.

Grains

Barley
Brown rice
(The longer you cook rice, the higher its glycemic response. Cook until just done.)
Buckwheat kasha
Bulgur
Couscous
Oat groats

Quinoa
Teff
Wheat berries

Dairy (Use in Moderation)
Buttermilk
Cheese (low-fat, low-sodium)
Cottage cheese (nonfat or low-fat)
Cream Cheese (nonfat or low-fat)
Parmesan cheese
Skim milk
Sour cream (nonfat)
Yogurt (nonfat, sugar-free)

Fats/Oils
Use monounsaturated and polyunsaturated fats only. Polyunsaturated oils should be expeller-pressed and stored in the refrigerator in dark, air-tight bottles.

Flaxseed oil (poly—should not be heated)
Hazelnut (mono)
Olive oil (mono—best for cooking)

Beverages
Club soda
Decaffeinated coffee (sweetened with acceptable sweetener)
Lemonade (homemade with xylitol or stevia)
Seltzer water (salt-free)
Tea (black, green, or herbal)
Tonic water (sugar-free)
Water

Meats, Poultry, Fish, and Eggs
Egg whites with an occasional yolk
Fish (salmon and other cold-water fish are best)
Poultry (skinless)
Shellfish

Sugars/Sweeteners
Brown rice syrup
Stevia
Xylitol

Miscellaneous
Catsup (Catsup is a high-glycemic food, but two to three
teaspoons on a turkey burger, for example, is okay)
Mustard
Salsa (sugar-free, no added corn syrup)
Soy sauce (low-sodium, small quantities)
Spices and herbs, fresh or dried

YOUR GUIDE TO EATING OUT

Restaurant food is notoriously high in salt and fat. However, restaurants are more accommodating than you might think. A National Restaurant Association survey found that close to 90 percent of all table-service restaurants will alter food preparation on request. Here's how to enjoy eating out while keeping with your program.

- Take the edge off your appetite by starting your meal with raw vegetables, a salad with low-fat dressing (on the side), or a light seafood appetizer.
- Choose entrees that are steamed, poached, broiled, roasted, baked, or cooked in their own juices. Fish is always an excellent choice. Pass on anything sautéed or fried.
- Avoid red meats. Remove the skin from your chicken or turkey before eating it.
- Avoid thick, creamy sauces such as hollandaise or bearnaise, or anything resembling gravy. Instead, choose stock-based or tomato-based sauces.
- Ask for your vegetables freshly steamed, with no added oil or butter.
- Order your salad dressing on the side or bring your own low-fat version. You might also try lemon juice or plain balsamic vinegar.

- Eat small or half-portion meals. You can always share, or take the rest home for another meal.

IN SUMMARY

This is the food plan I recommend for my patients with hypertension. In fact, it is pretty much what I recommend for all my patients, and it's the type of food served at the Whitaker Wellness Institute in Newport Beach, California. To help you get started, in Appendix C I've offered some suggested menus for two weeks and included recipes for several of the dishes. These are tasty, not unduly restrictive menus that you should be able to stick with. Once you become familiar with the types of foods and see how they are prepared, you'll be ready to branch out on your own. The idea isn't to throw out everything you like and are used to eating, but to learn how to modify your favorite dishes and make them healthier. (Unfortunately, I haven't found a way to make prime rib healthier!) Remember, this isn't a quick fix but a lifelong way of eating to engender optimal health and normal blood pressure.

Patients sometimes ask me if they have to eat like this forever. This is a reasonable question. Some of you will respond quickly to the measures suggested in this book, others more slowly. For some, exercise will make up for dietary indiscretions, but for others dietary slips will make a real difference in blood pressure control. You're going to have to give it the old college try—I recommend strict compliance for at least a month—and then see what sort of give-and-take your body can handle. None of us are perfect. We all "fall off the wagon" from time to time. What is important is that you get back on. Remember, this isn't a quick fix. It's a food plan to follow over a lifetime.

CHAPTER 12

The Hypertension-Water Connection

William, a retired army colonel, had been on calcium channel blockers and diuretics to control his high blood pressure for years. He read about a revolutionary way of lowering blood pressure: simply drinking adequate amounts of water. Although he was dubious, the case for this therapy was convincing, and William decided to give it a try. He gradually stopped taking his medications and at the same time began drinking a minimum of eight 8-ounce glasses of water every day. He didn't change his diet or exercise pattern—he just started drinking more water. When William first got off his antihypertensive medications, his blood pressure climbed to 150–160/95–98 mm Hg. However, as he continued on his new program of increased water it gradually began to drop. He faithfully monitored his blood pressure every day, and over the next three months it averaged 130–135/75–80 mm Hg. William remains drug-free, and his blood pressure continues to be in the normal range—all because he began drinking adequate amounts of water.

This chapter will radically change the way you think about water. In medical school I was taught that water was a relatively inert substance in the body. Even though water accounts for over half of our body mass, its vital role in human health was never properly addressed. It was simply there. Somewhere along the way it dawned on me that a substance that comprises over 50 percent of the finely engineered human organism surely must have unique, undiscovered properties. After all, next to oxygen it is our most essential requirement for life.

The human body is a water-based environment. Every single biological function depends upon the efficient flow of water. It is the universal solvent in which a variety of vital solutes are dissolved. It is the aqueous portion of the blood *(plasma)* and the fluid both inside cells *(intracellular fluid)* and outside them *(extracellular fluid)*. Water is necessary for the distribution of nutrients throughout the body and the removal of waste products from the cells. It is intimately involved in your body's acid-base balance, and it is the medium through which hormones and other chemical messengers travel. Water is an important component of skin, cartilage, and other tissues, and it helps maintain body temperature. Furthermore, it acts as a shuttle for the electrolytic minerals such as sodium and potassium that fuel your cells' all-important electrical activity, as discussed in Chapter 8.

The exact amount of water contained within your body depends on the balance between your fluid intake and excretion. You derive water from three sources: drink (60 percent), food (30 percent), and cellular metabolism, or oxidation (10 percent). At the same time, you constantly lose water—primarily through the lungs and skin (36 percent), and urine (60 percent). Some is lost in the stool as well. Hot weather, physical activity, and illness that involves diarrhea and vomiting also influence water balance. Given all the important roles water plays in your body, it is obvious that being adequately hydrated is essential for health. The best way to remain hydrated is to drink lots of water. If you do not, you're heading for trouble.

THE HAZARDS OF DEHYDRATION

If you are shorting yourself on water, you're making yourself sick. In his book *Your Body's Many Cries for Water*, F. Batmanghelidj, M.D., proposes a paradigm-shifting theory: Chronic, unintentional dehydration is the root of many of our serious maladies, including asthma, arthritis, lower back pain, and hypertension.

Your body maintains its fluid volume by a system of electrolytic mineral exchange in and out of your body's cells. The mineral central

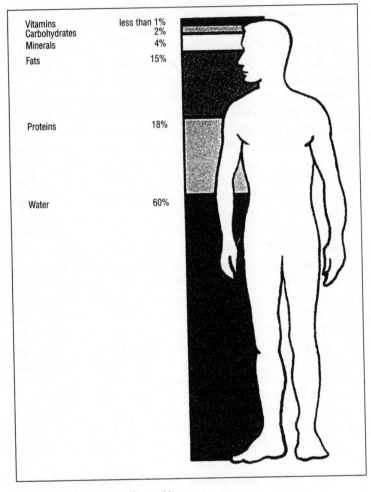

Vitamins	less than 1%
Carbohydrates	2%
Minerals	4%
Fats	15%
Proteins	18%
Water	60%

Figure 9. Your Body's Water Composition

to this, as you might suspect from our discussions in previous chapters, is sodium. When water volume is suboptimal, the kidneys reabsorb more sodium, which is followed by a rise in fluid levels in the body. Because adequate hydration is so important, the body is remarkably efficient at maintaining water balance.

If fluid losses are too great or water intake chronically deficient, however, your body makes adjustments to maintain fluid and blood flow to the areas most crucial for life. Blood is shunted from less essential tissues in the peripheral areas so that the brain, heart, and other vital organs continue to receive enough to meet their basic needs. As we discussed in Chapter 2, blood flow is diverted by constriction of the arterioles. And this at the same time decreases the diameter of the "pipes" and raises blood pressure. It also results in a shutting down of some capillaries. The longer the body is in a dehydrated state, the more prolonged the absence of blood to the tissues these capillaries supply. Bereft of adequate nutrients and bogged down with cellular wastes, these tissues are unable to function properly. Dr. Batmanghelidj has proposed this mechanism as being a primary contributor to a host of medical problems.

ANOTHER REASON TO AVOID DIURETICS

This understanding of how dehydration contributes to high blood pressure forces us to look at diuretics, the most popular drug treatment for hypertension, in a new light. Physicians prescribe diuretics to reduce the pressure caused by "too much fluid in the pipes." But if hypertension is—if only in part—caused or exacerbated by chronic water shortage, diuretics, which cause *more* water loss, will only aggravate the condition and make the body even more determined to hold on to sodium in an effort to maintain its water reserves.

Diuretic drugs, as noted in Chapter 7, force the kidneys to excrete more sodium in the urine, and it takes with it water and water-soluble nutrients that play a key role in regulating blood pressure. The nutrient losses caused by these drugs affect not only your blood pressure, but tissues throughout your body. I often wonder about the extent of the damage caused by this myopic approach to hypertension. Some people, quite logically, are concerned that drinking too much water will increase their fluid levels and, therefore, their blood pressure. As contradictory as it may sound, the truth is that water is a powerful diuretic—the best diuretic! The more water you drink, the more fluid your kidneys excrete as urine. Capillaries open since there is less need to conserve water, resistance on the peripheral blood vessels decreases, and blood pressure goes down. Over time, as William's story illustrates, water can even replace the need for medication.

MAKE SURE YOU DRINK ENOUGH WATER

Most of us don't drink enough water. Sure, we'll load up when we're thirsty, but few of us keep track of how much we really drink. We just take it for granted that we get enough. Well, you probably don't. The thirst mechanism, which is controlled by an area in the hypothalamus of the brain called the thirst center, kicks in when there is a decrease in water volume, but thirst is quenched as soon as you start drinking water. During hot weather and especially during athletic endeavors, your thirst may be quenched long before you've had adequate water. Furthermore, many people, particularly the elderly, either do not recognize or ignore thirst signals. To get enough water you must *conscientiously* drink eight to ten 8-ounce glasses of water per day. If you have hypertension, your ultimate goal should be ten to twelve 8-ounce glasses, or 96 ounces of water per day.

This may seem like a lot, but remember, you are rehydrating yourself. We naturally lose an average of 2½ quarts of water per day. As I mentioned above, urination, sweat, and respiration are all natural processes that result in water loss. We also lose extra water under special circumstances, such as fever, diarrhea, kidney disease, or diabetes. Drinking alcohol or coffee, tea, and other caffeinated beverages causes further dehydration, increasing your need for water replacement. Some experts maintain that for every cup of caffeine-containing beverages you drink, you should drink an extra cup of water to make up for the water loss prompted by caffeine.

Although I want you to drink sufficient water, I don't want you to go overboard. Drinking too much water—more than the 96 ounces per day I recommend—can stress your kidneys and digestive system. Hypertension, diabetes, and stress all leave the kidneys in a weakened state, so be careful. In fact, if you have kidney disease or congestive heart disease, consult your physician before increasing your water intake.

Also, keep in mind that, much like a sponge, your body can absorb water only at a limited rate. It will require some time to adapt to your new level of intake. So when you begin your rehydration program, step up your water intake gradually. As you cut back on dehydrating beverages such as coffee and alcohol, you should increase your water intake by about a cup a day until you reach your goal. Don't forget that you need to drink more when you exercise—the Mayo Clinic recommends two to three glasses of water before exercise and 4 to 6 ounces every 10 to 15 minutes during strenuous workouts.

Because water intake is such an important part of this program, I've come up with a few tips on how to get all that water down. The best overall approach to rehydration is to have a tall glass of water when you wake up and another glass every hour or so through the day. Keep filled water bottles in your car, at your desk, and anywhere else you spend time. Finally, remember to keep a glass of water next to your bed in case you wake up thirsty during the night. This should enable you to reach your ten- to twelve-cup goal. The most common complaint I hear from patients trying to follow this routine is that they often feel full and bloated before their first glass is even finished. This is partially due to the fact that when you swallow water, you also swallow air—that's what makes the gulping sound you hear as you drink it down. A simple solution to this problem is to drink water through a straw. You'll consume much less air (four to five times less), feel less full, and find it easier to get your daily quota.

MAKE SURE YOUR WATER IS CLEAN

It's no secret that our municipal tap water is less than pristine. According to Environmental Protection Agency (EPA) records, from 1971 through 1990 there were 570 documented cases in this country of contaminated water causing illnesses affecting thousands of people. The Centers for Disease Control (CDC) estimate that more than a million people every year get sick from microorganisms in drinking water, and 900 to 1,000 die as a result! City water is heavily chlorinated to kill germs. Although this has slashed the incidence of waterborne diseases, chlorination of our water supplies has created an unanticipated, largely unrecognized problem. Chlorine reacts with organic substances such as decaying vegetation in water to create by-products known as *halogenated organic compounds,* or *tri-halomethanes,* such as chloroform. These chlorine breakdown products have been implicated in cancers of the bladder, colon, and rectum, as well as in miscarriages.

City water is also fluoridated to prevent tooth decay, and some cities add calcium hydroxide or other alkaline substances to change the pH (acidity) of the water so it doesn't corrode pipes. In addition, heavy metals, including copper and lead, both of which are linked to hypertension and other health problems, have been found in tap water. In 1993 the EPA identified more than 800 water systems, supplying some 30 million Americans, with levels of lead in excess of recommended guidelines. But even if water is lead-free when it leaves the treatment facility, lead may leach out from lead pipes, which are common in older buildings, or lead-soldered pipe joints, which were used until the late 1980s.

My point is that the quality of the water you drink is of paramount importance. You need to drink pure water to get well. Bottled water is an option, but it is expensive, poorly regulated, and, according to some surveys, sometimes little better than tap water. To play it safe, you should consider investing in a home water-treatment system that will consistently maintain the quality of your drinking water. The economics of home filtering are also far more advantageous than buying bottled water. In general, tap water costs about one-tenth of a cent per gallon, while a well-maintained filter unit delivers water at about 5 cents per gallon. Bottled water, however, costs up to $1.60 per gallon, and often the water you're buying is filtered with technology that you could have in your own home.

Some home water-treatment systems, like the sink-side plastic pitchers with replaceable filters, are inexpensive but do little more than reduce the chlorine taste and some of the minerals. I don't recommend reverse-osmosis systems or distillers, because they remove magnesium, calcium, and important trace minerals that are important for blood pressure control. Furthermore, these systems do not remove chlorination by-products unless used in conjunction with another type of filtration. In my opinion, the best water-treatment systems combine an activated solid carbon block filter with an ultraviolet (UV) light chamber. The carbon filter improves taste and removes chemical and organic pollutants and chlorination by-products, while the UV chamber kills microbes in the water.

The unique water-treatment system that I use in my home and office is the Sun-Pure. It has two separate filters for removing harmful impurities, including chlorine, rust, radon, sediment, aluminum, lead, and disease-causing organisms. But more important, it's the only home-based water purifier I know of that uses ultraviolet light to remove disease-causing pathogens, bacteria, and viruses (filtration alone doesn't do this). Sun-Pure is so good that Faith Baptist missionaries from Indiana use it in areas of Central America and Mexico where cholera is prevalent to transform swamp water into crystal-clear drinking water.

IN SUMMARY

1. Hydrate your body with 96 ounces (ten to twelve 8-ounce glasses) of water per day. Build up to this slowly. If you have kidney disease or congestive heart failure, consult your doctor before increasing your water intake dramatically.
2. Drink extra water when you exercise—two or three glasses before you exercise and 4 to 6 ounces every 10 to 15 minutes during workouts.
3. If drinking water from a glass makes you feel bloated or full, drink through a straw instead.
4. Purify the water you drink with a home filtration system. The one I use both at home and in my office is the Sun-Pure water purifier. See Appendix E for ordering information.

CHAPTER 13

Exercise Your Way to Healthier Blood Pressure

In his thirties and forties Nick was an active man who enjoyed tennis, swimming, and golf and worked at a physically demanding job. In his fifties he switched to a desk job and began exercising less frequently, and by the time he retired, he had given up most physical activity. His blood pressure was a high 172/98, even with medication. When Nick experienced a ministroke at the age of 68, he took it as a wake-up call to get moving.

He signed up for a program of cardiac rehabilitation at his local hospital, where he learned how to exercise safely and monitor his heart rate. Three times a week he walked on a treadmill for 20 minutes, then worked out on weight machines to strengthen his muscles. By the end of the three-month period, his blood pressure was down to 140/70. More important, his energy, his mood—in fact, his whole attitude toward life—had improved so much that he signed on at the hospital gym as a regular member.

The benefits of exercise are enormous, and if you have high blood pressure, it just might save your life. Regular exercise strengthens the heart and helps normalize blood pressure. Because it increases insulin sensitivity and stabilizes blood-glucose levels, it is one of the most effective therapies for insulin resistance, which is often a precursor to hypertension. Exercise also improves the ratio of body fat to lean muscle mass and promotes weight loss. Furthermore, it has also been shown to raise levels of protective HDL cholesterol and to normalize the heart's electrical activity. Regular exercise significantly reduces the risk of atherosclerosis and hypertension—and these are only its heart-related benefits.

Exercise also restores your metabolism to youthful levels, strengthens your bones, and prevents muscle atrophy. It improves your mood, your mental functioning, and your sex drive. With all of the known benefits of exercise, I often wonder why so few Americans exercise on a regular basis. I'm sure I've heard all of the excuses—from lack of time to fatigue to overwhelming laziness. But think about it. Isn't it worth a few hours a week to gain all of the important health improvements associated with exercise?

HOW EXERCISE REDUCES BLOOD PRESSURE

Hundreds of studies have demonstrated that regular exercise reduces blood pressure and lowers the incidence of heart disease. Exercise improves blood flow and encourages the capillary beds in the muscles and other tissues to open. This places less resistance on the arteries and arterioles and lowers blood pressure. Exercise also improves the elasticity and responsiveness of the arteries and reduces the risk of atherosclerosis, other important factors in blood pressure control. Furthermore, as I will describe below, exercise significantly enhances the muscles' insulin sensitivity, which is a factor in many cases of hypertension.

An Australian research team reviewed and analyzed twenty-nine studies on the effects of exercise on blood pressure in order to identify the optimal type, intensity, and frequency of exercise for managing hypertension. They included in their analysis only randomized, controlled trials that lasted at least four weeks. These twenty-nine studies involved 1,533 hypertensive and normotensive participants, and the bulk of them examined the effects of aerobic exercise training. The researchers found that aerobic exercise reduced systolic blood pressure by an average of 4.7 mm Hg and diastolic blood pressure by an average of 3.1 mm Hg, compared with nonexercising control groups. These reductions in blood pressure with aerobic exercise were independent of the exercise intensity; that is, working out at a high intensity was no more effective than moderate-intensity exercise. Furthermore, this study found no advantage to exercising more than three times a week.

Other studies have confirmed the blood-pressure-reducing effects of less-intense exercise. In a 1999 study conducted at the Welch Center for Prevention, Epidemiology, and Clinical Research, Johns Hopkins Medical Institutions, in Baltimore, 62 inactive adults 60 years of age or older with high blood pressure but not on medications were enrolled in a twelve-week program of exercise. They were instructed to do either moderate-intensity aerobic exercise or Tai Chi, a form of low-intensity exercise involving slow, fluid, and continuous movements that rarely speed up heart rate. The goal for both the Tai Chi and the aerobic groups was to exercise 30 minutes a day, four days per week. After twelve weeks systolic and diastolic blood pressures fell in both groups, with no significant differences between the two groups. Based on these and other studies, it appears that over the long term, low-intensity training may do as much, if not more, to lower blood pressure than moderate- or high-intensity training. This is excellent news. It means you don't have to run marathons or compete in triathlons. A regular, sustained low-intensity walking program is perfectly adequate.

Exercise may take some time to do its magic, as a study published in the *American Journal of Cardiology* attests. In this study, 60- to 69-year-olds with essential hypertension exercised at either low or moderate intensity. After nine months with this exercise program, systolic blood pressure decreased a total of 20 mm Hg in the low-intensity group and only 8 mm Hg in the moderate-intensity group. Both groups exhibited between 11 and 12 mm Hg reductions in diastolic blood pressure.

Beyond its benefits for hypertension, exercise diminishes cardiovascular risk factors and significantly reduces death rates from all causes—which is what hypertension control is all about in the first place. Two studies published in the *New England Journal of Medicine* confirmed this. In the first of these studies, 1,960 healthy men ages 40 to 59 were divided into four groups according to their level of physical activity and were followed for sixteen years. At the end of this period, the rate of death from heart disease in the least active group was four times higher than in the most active group. In addition, physical activity reduced deaths from all other causes, not just heart disease. Rather than simply saying that exercise is protective, this research suggests that inactivity is a risk factor in itself for heart attack and premature death.

The second study was an interim report on the long-term evaluation of 10,269 Harvard University men who have been tracked periodically since 1962. Again, the benefits of physical activity were obvious. The men who engaged in moderately vigorous physical exercise experienced a 41 percent lower risk of death from heart disease, as well as a 23 percent reduction in all causes of death, compared with men who were inactive. The conclusions were the same as those in the first study. Not only does physical activity reduce death rates, inactivity increases risk of death.

EXERCISE IMPROVES INSULIN RESISTANCE

Regular physical activity is also an important factor in improving insulin resistance, as it markedly enhances insulin sensitivity and glucose uptake in the skeletal muscles. This relationship has been confirmed in numerous studies, including a recent clinical trial performed in Sweden. In this study, younger people exhibited improved insulin sensitivity after only a single exercise session. The same effect is possible in middle-aged or older individuals after just a few training sessions and can last for as long as three to six days. I find this remarkable! One or two days of exercise can improve your insulin sensitivity for nearly a week!

This same study showed that aerobic and resistance exercise, or strength training, were effective in enhancing insulin sensitivity. The authors of the study explained that exercise may stimulate the release of certain sex hormones, which in turn facilitate the insulin response. Exercise also increases the levels of a glucose-transport protein called GLUT-4, improves glycogen uptake, and increases the activity of the muscle capillary network. This means that as long as you continue to work out consistently, you will steadily improve your body's response to insulin, perhaps even gradually reversing all of the variables of syndrome X, discussed in Chapter 6. Your body fat and body mass index (BMI) will begin to come down, your blood glucose levels will normalize, your HDL cholesterol will rise, and your blood pressure will gradually fall. Quite simply, regular exercise can literally give you a second chance at good health.

DON'T FEAR EXERCISE-INDUCED HYPERTENSION

Some patients with hypertension are afraid to exercise, fearing that exercise will increase their blood pressure and precipitate a heart attack or stroke. This is understandable, especially in light of the occasional much-publicized sudden deaths of healthy-appearing serious exercisers. I am often asked about running guru Jim Fixx, one of the early proponents of jogging, who regularly ran sixty miles a week. When he dropped dead one day at the end of a four-mile run, many jogging enthusiasts, especially heart patients and their doctors, questioned the safety of exercise. What most people don't know is what Fixx's autopsy revealed. Fixx not only had three coronary arteries that were almost completely blocked, he also had scar tissue from previous heart attacks on three areas of his heart, one of which had occurred only about two weeks before he died. Jim Fixx also had a congenital heart condition called biventricular hypertrophy, which causes the heart to become abnormally enlarged. My point is that Fixx was overdoing it for a man with these conditions. I am not asking you to run sixty miles a week. I am simply suggesting you pick up an activity you enjoy and make sure you get moving several times a week. Yes, exercise does increase your blood pressure temporarily. But only *while* you're exercising. Your reward will be a lasting reduction in blood pressure *after* the exercise.

One large-scale study that may put you at ease demonstrates that the exaggerated systolic blood pressure elevation response to exercise (which is what exercise hypertension is) is a desirable effect. Of the 9,608 adults who were evaluated by treadmill testing, those *with* exercise hypertension had a lower likelihood of coronary heart disease and lower death rates. In other words, coronary disease and death were less common in those who experienced a rise in their systolic blood pressure when exercising—the very thing many hypertensive patients fear.

If you have been inactive, I strongly recommend that you take an *exercise stress test* before you begin your new exercise program. This simple, painless procedure is usually conducted on a treadmill or stationary bicycle in your doctor's office. While you exercise, several monitors will measure your vital signs. Your physician will then use this information, which includes an electrocardiogram (EKG), to determine your fitness level. The test uncovers any abnormalities that could occur during physical activity, including arrhythmias, skipped heartbeats, or a limited ability to take in oxygen. Testing could also reveal poor circulation to sections of the heart, which would turn exercise from friend to foe. A stress test is especially important if you smoke, have high cholesterol, or are over age 45. After the test, your physician will be able to give you specific guidelines, including exercise activities and intensity levels that will allow you to exercise safely and derive maximum benefit from your efforts.

DESIGN YOUR OWN PERSONALIZED EXERCISE PROGRAM

The key is to increase your physical endurance by doing something healthy, fun, and physical for 30 minutes, four to five times per week. Aim for regular, not rigorous, exercise. It's better to be gentle and consistent rather than strenuous and sporadic. Routine low- and moderate-intensity exercise will give you the greatest health benefits, so pace yourself and work up gradually to your exercise goal. Remember, exercising for 30 minutes four or five times per week is your *goal*—it's not where you begin. Start slowly with something you enjoy, whether it's a walk around the block or a bike ride through the neighborhood. Bodies come in different shapes and sizes and have different capabilities, so choose something fun and go at your own pace. Do not, I repeat, *DO NOT* be a weekend warrior. People who engage in sporadic high-intensity exercise are only looking for trouble. Instead, choose moderate activities such as those suggested below that you can commit to on a regular basis.

The focus of this chapter is on aerobic exercise, the kind that gets your heart rate up and delivers more oxygen to the heart and muscles. Virtually all of the studies demonstrating the benefits of exercise on cardiovascular health, including the above-mentioned studies on lowering blood pressure, have utilized aerobic exercise. This is not to ignore the two other major types of exercise, weight training and stretching. Both have significant health benefits, and I frequently recommend them to my patients. However, since aerobic exercise is most directly related to lowering blood pressure, that is what we will concentrate on.

 RECOMMENDED EXERCISE ACTIVITIES

- Aerobics
- Bicycling
- Circuit weight training
- Dancing
- Jazzercize
- Jogging
- Racquetball
- Squash
- Swimming
- Tai chi
- Tennis
- Walking

Whatever exercise you choose, make sure you keep it at a low to moderate level of intensity. One way to make sure you are in this range is to listen to your body. You should feel exertion, but not to the point of exhaustion or pain. You should be able to carry on a conversation while exercising at this intensity. Another way to monitor your level of activity is by taking your pulse periodically while you exercise. Here's how:

1. Place your middle and index fingers either on the side of your neck or inside of your wrist, below your thumb. Find your pulse and count the number of beats you feel during a six-second time frame.

2. Add a zero to your six-second pulse count to get a rough estimate of your heart rate per minute.

3. Keep your heart rate within your target range (see the table below). If your heart rate is higher than your maximum target, slow down. However, if it is consistently lower than the recommended minimum heart rate for your age, you need to increase your exercise intensity. Only when your heart rate reaches this minimum level are you bringing in enough oxygen to the muscles and the heart to achieve the benefits of aerobic exercise. An exception, however, appears to be Tai chi, which has been demonstrated to effectively lower blood pressure.

▼ TARGET RANGES FOR EXERCISING HEART RATE

Your Age	Minimum Heart Rate	Maximum Heart Rate	10-Second Pulse (minimum–maximum)
20–29	120	151	20–25
30–39	114	143	19–24
40–49	108	135	18–22
50–59	102	127	17–21
60–69	96	120	16–20
70+	90	112	15–19

HOW TO BEGIN A WALKING PROGRAM

I play squash several times a week and cycle occasionally, but among my favorite exercise activities is walking with my wife and dogs. It doesn't require a lot of equipment—just a pair of good running or walking shoes. It doesn't take a lot of time either. Rather than driving to the gym, we just round up our dogs, Fritz and Lacy, step out the front door, head out for 15 minutes in one direction, then turn around and come back. It can be done most anywhere, making it an ideal activity to keep up while traveling. In fact, it's a great way to see new areas. For us, it's also a chance to get out by ourselves for a brief time, away from the kids, and just talk. For most people, particularly those of you who have been inactive, walking is the ideal form of exercise.

Walking is an aerobic workout that transports oxygen into your body while stimulating your large muscle groups. When you walk at a healthy, moderate pace, oxygen circulates to every neglected crevice and corner of your body. With a regular walking program, your muscle mass increases and body fat decreases, leading to weight loss and an improved BMI. HDL cholesterol rises, improving your cardiovascular health. Endorphins are released and your mood lifts. Because walking is a weight-bearing exercise, your bones become stronger. Insulin sensitivity is heightened, and blood pressure falls. All of these benefits just from regular walking!

Here are a few simple tips to help you get started on a successful walking program:

- Get a good pair of walking or running shoes. You don't have to spend $100 on a pair endorsed by a famous athlete; the most expensive and gimmicky aren't necessarily the best. Shop around and try on a few different brands. If you haven't bought a pair of walking or running shoes in a while, you'll be amazed at how comfortable and supportive shoes are these days. Don't forget to break them in by wearing them around the house for a few hours before you go on your first walk.
- Wear comfortable clothing. You don't need anything fancy, just loose apparel that breathes. Cotton is always a good choice. And if you're in a cold climate, layer your clothes for warmth.
- Pick a safe, scenic walking route. Plan where you are going. Steer clear of busy traffic areas, but also stay away from isolated areas if they make you uncomfortable. When you're walking in a new city on a trip, make sure the surrounding area is safe for walkers before you head out.
- Stretch out for about five minutes before you begin walking. It's

critical to warm your muscles before a workout so you won't injure yourself. Even the smallest stretching effort will bring big rewards. Try side stretches, neck stretches, shoulder rolls, calf stretches, hamstring stretches, and inner-thigh stretches.

- Drink a glass or two of water before you begin so you're well hydrated for your walking workout, and drink more when you finish.
- Go at your own pace. You're not in competition with anyone, including yourself.
- Pump your arms as you walk if you want to increase intensity.
- Walk tall. Walk with purpose. Think about how wonderful this exercise is for your mind and your body.
- When you're done walking, do another five minutes of cooldown stretches. This will improve your flexibility and give your body a chance to return to its resting state.
- If you've been inactive up to now, begin your walking program slowly and build up. Here is a suggested schedule for getting started:

    Week 1—Walk for 10 minutes four times a week.

    Week 2—Walk for 15 minutes four times a week.

    Week 3—Walk for 20 minutes four or five times a week.

    Week 4—Walk for 25 minutes four or five times a week.

    Week 5—Walk for 30 minutes four or five times a week.

Monitor your intensity by checking your pulse, per the instructions on page 181. Again, don't exceed your maximum target heart rate, but if you are below the minimum rate, step up your pace. You'll find that as you progress, your speed will pick up and you'll be able to walk farther and faster during your 30-minute workout. If you want to increase your efforts, build up to a maximum of 45 to 60 minutes. But exercise no more than six days a week; your body needs at least one day of rest.

▼ | STRETCHING

The general purpose of stretching is to prepare the body for more vigorous levels of activity and reduce the likelihood of injuring yourself while exercising.

Stretching should immediately follow the warm-up period. It should be done slowly, holding each stretch for 15–30 seconds. You should go just to the point of tightness, to be able to "feel the stretch." Never force it or bounce during a particular stretching exercise. When the muscle is stretched too fast, it reacts by tightening slightly to protect itself from tearing, causing it to become tighter than it was when you began the stretch.

Stretching briefly after exercise lessens the likelihood of delayed muscle soreness and reduced joint mobility.

These stretches were prepared by Whitaker Wellness Institute exercise physiologist, Dr. Daren Gregson.

To stretch all of your major muscle groups, perform these 9 stretches. Stretch to your own personal point of tightness, and hold each stretch for about 30 seconds, then relax. If a stretch involves movement to one side, make sure to repeat it on the other side.

1. Full-body stretch

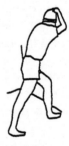

2. Calf stretch

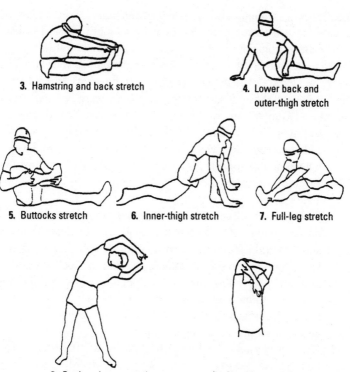

3. Hamstring and back stretch

4. Lower back and outer-thigh stretch

5. Buttocks stretch

6. Inner-thigh stretch

7. Full-leg stretch

8. Back and arm stretch

9. Shoulder stretch

HOW TO MAKE EXERCISE A PART OF YOUR LIFE

Despite all of the well-known benefits of exercise, the U.S. surgeon general and the American College of Sports Medicine report that fewer than 10 percent of Americans exercise at the recommended level, and as many as 30 percent don't exercise at all! Considering the importance of exercise for good health, these are appalling statistics. It's not lack of knowledge that keeps people from exercising—even you couch potatoes know it's good for you—it's just human nature. Most people avoid physical activity unless it's a necessary component in their life. In the not-so-distant past, physical activity was a part of everyday life. People didn't jump in the car to drive two blocks to the grocery store; they walked. They likely grew at least part of the food they ate, which required tilling, weeding, and other labors. Today it is possible to live most of your life exerting no more physical activity than walking from your home to your car and to an elevator.

What can you do to make exercise a regular part of your life? Is it discipline, guilt, or the natural inclination to do what's best for you? No, it's none of these. If any of these motivators were successful, you would have traded your easy chair for a bicycle long ago. To stay active and physically fit and to enjoy the fruits of your physical activity, you need to change the way you think about exercise and to develop and implement a reasonable exercise program. It's not hard. Just follow these recommendations:

1. Change your attitude. Exercise is not just something you should do for your health. It's life-affirming! It's fun! Start thinking about it in these positive terms, rather than as something you know you need to do but don't really want to. Look at exercise as a mind-expanding, mood-elevating, longevity-producing experience. Know that as you exercise, you are lowering your blood pressure and getting healthier. You can live without exercise, but not nearly as long or as well.

2. Copy the exercise log I've provided (Figure 10) and use it to help you commit to and accomplish your goals. The log is set up to track your exercise activities over a one-week period. Take a few moments at the beginning of the week to plan your exercise schedule. Commit yourself—in writing—to specific days, times, and activities. Strive for at least 30 minutes of exercise four times per week. Check the "Done!" box whenever you complete your planned activity. If you don't get around to your planned activity on one day, try to make it up another day that week. Use the log to track how your activities make you *feel,* both physically and mentally. You'll be amazed at the improvements you'll experience on both counts.

3. Get a friend to participate in your new regimen. You'll find it's much easier to get moving when there is someone waiting at your front door to exercise with you. It's more fun, too.

4. Set specific goals for individual feats. For instance, one summer a few years ago I fulfilled a lifelong goal of bicycling across the

country. We dipped our wheels in the Pacific Ocean in Washington State, and ten weeks later we dipped them into the Potomac River in Washington, D.C. Now, I'm not recommending that you undertake such an endeavor—there were times when I wondered why in the world I did! But the point is, knowing that I would be cycling up to 100 miles a day a few months down the line made it easier for me to get out and train. I knew I'd pay the price if I wasn't in shape. I've done other exercise feats that required regular training. A couple of years ago, five of my buddies and I signed up for a 10-kilometer obstacle course at a nearby Marine base. "The Dirty Half-Dozen" jumped over hedges and waded through mud pits. We didn't set any records, but we finished and had a blast. And for several months leading up to the race, I was motivated to get out and run several times a week. My point is that without these commitments, I would have been much more sedentary. With these commitments, however, I felt motivated to stick with my exercise program. If you've chosen walking as your workout, consider entering a community-sponsored or fund-raising 5-kilometer run/walk. A few weeks of training will prepare you for this 3.2-mile race, and you'll have a goal to work toward.

IN SUMMARY

1. If you have been inactive, and especially if you are over age 45 or have any chronic illnesses, check with your doctor before beginning an exercise program.
2. Set exercise goals—aim for at least 30 minutes four or five times a week—and stick with them. You may build up to 60 minutes up to six days a week.
3. Warm up and cool down by stretching for five minutes before and five minutes after exercise.
4. Stay within your target heart rate, according to the chart on page 181. Listen to your body and don't overdo it.
5. Drink a cup or two of water before and after exercising. If your workout is prolonged, don't forget to drink even more often.

Exercise Log Week of __/__/__ to __/__/__

Day of Week	Activity	Exercise Time	Done!	How I Feel
Monday			☐	
Tuesday			☐	
Wednesday			☐	
Thursday			☐	
Friday			☐	
Saturday			☐	
Sunday				
Comments:				

Figure 10. Exercise Log

CHAPTER 14

Reduce the Stress in Your Life—and Your Blood Pressure

Allison is a petite, vivacious woman who looks at least ten years younger than her sixty-nine years. She works out at a gym several times a week, watches what she eats, and is on a good nutritional supplement program. Although she has never had any serious health problems, several months ago she began feeling tired, anxious, and out of sorts. She admitted that she was under a lot of stress. She had remarried the previous year after thirty years of living on her own, and although she loves Ed, the adjustment was much harder than either of them anticipated. Their communication styles just didn't mesh. If there was a problem, Allison wanted to talk about it and clear it up, while Ed would just clam up and refuse to even admit anything was wrong. As the months wore on, Allison became increasingly frustrated and unhappy.

When Allison went in for her yearly checkup, she was shocked to learn that her blood pressure was an alarming 200/100. Follow-up visits to her doctor confirmed the diagnosis of hypertension, and she was prescribed a beta-blocker. Yet even on the drug her blood pressure remained high. Allison knew there was a link between her high blood pressure and her situation at home. She confronted Ed and finally made him understand that she could not live with the underlying stress in their relationship. Ed told her that he would do his best to improve his communication skills. Things didn't get dramatically better overnight, but Ed did begin to talk more and share his feelings, and Allison gradually began to feel as if she were again in control of her life. After another month, her blood pressure returned to normal.

You know that lack of exercise, an improper diet, and nutritional deficiencies can raise blood pressure. But marital discord? Constant financial worries? Problems with your boss or coworkers? Sure, these and other upsets get us riled up, but can they really cause chronic elevations in blood pressure? Absolutely! Dozens of epidemiological studies have found correlations between hypertension and the stressors of daily living. Physicians reported that during World War II, citizens in the besieged city of Leningrad tended to have above-normal blood pressure. High rates of hypertension are observed in individuals in developing countries who are forced to trade their traditional way of life for city living. In the United States, blacks and whites alike with low socioeconomic status have higher than average blood pressure. And a 1999 study showed that an unhappy marriage can raise blood pressure.

It is well established that chronic anxiety and stress play a significant role in hypertension. Noted Harvard University professor Herbert Benson, M.D., in his book *The Relaxation Response,* suggests that stress might underlie the 90 to 95 percent of all cases of hypertension that are classified as being of "unknown cause." As I explained in Chapter 2, the sympathetic nervous system has a profound impact on blood pressure, and one way in which it elevates blood pressure is the stress response.

HOW STRESS RAISES BLOOD PRESSURE

The stress response, also called the *general adaptation syndrome,* is a physiological reaction that rallies you to action when you encounter a perceived threat. It is a natural protective mechanism that evolved eons ago, when the proper response to most of mankind's threats— wild animals, warring tribes, and natural disasters—was to run or fight. This "fight-or-flight" response gets you ready for action. It begins in the hypothalamus, an area of the brain that regulates many of our involuntary functions and is intimately involved in basic survival.

The hypothalamus signals the adjacent pituitary gland to secrete a hormone that activates the adrenal glands to release epinephrine (also called adrenaline) and norepinephrine (or noradrenaline). These stress hormones speed up your heart rate, and you begin to breathe faster. To ready you for physical action, your arteries constrict and extra blood is diverted to your muscles. Your brain is flooded with chemicals that make you alert and on guard. Digestive processes take a backseat as blood is shunted from the stomach. A rush of glucose is emptied into your bloodstream for extra energy. This is known as the *alarm reaction* phase of the stress response.

Once the threat is past, systems return to normal and stress hormone levels—and blood pressure—fall. However, if stress is chronic, a second stage, known as *resistance reaction*, sets in. Other adrenal hormones, called *glucocorticoids* or *corticosteroids*, are secreted, and additional biochemical changes take place as your body continues to be on the alert. Your body eventually becomes depleted of magnesium, potassium, and other nutrients essential for blood pressure control, and blood pressure remains elevated. The final stage of the stress response is *exhaustion*. Adrenal hormone stores are depleted, and organ systems begin to fail.

Logically, of course, you can sort out which perceived threats require springing into action and which ones should be dealt with in more appropriate ways. In twenty-first-century America you may occasionally require the physical readiness that the stress response activates. But the vast majority of your stressors are likely to be emotional or psychological threats for which the fight-or-flight response is unnecessary. Unfortunately, your body cannot differentiate between physical and psychological, so you are subjected to this entire physiological response each time you perceive a threat, even if it is just emotional distress. When this happens repeatedly, your body begins to suffer the effects of chronic stress. Your muscles remain tense, which may result in backache or "a pain in the neck." You might have digestive repercussions—your emotional problems might "give you an ulcer." Or your problems might "raise your blood pressure." It's no accident that these expressions have crept into our speech to describe the effects of stress.

CHRONIC STRESS AND HYPERTENSION

The links between hypertension and stress have been addressed in hundreds of studies. Anxiety, anger—particularly repressed anger—depression, feelings of lack of control, defensiveness, even marital discord have all been demonstrated to contribute to elevated blood pressure. A 1997 study published in the *Archives of Family Medicine* linked both anxiety and depression to an increased risk of hypertension. Researchers followed 2,992 volunteers who had no initial signs of hypertension for seven to sixteen years and regularly assessed their levels of anxiety and depression using standard psychological tests. At the conclusion of the study, it became evident that those who were the most anxious or depressed were at greater risk of developing hypertension, and the risk was even more pronounced for blacks than it was for whites.

One concept I find particularly intriguing is that stress originates not from the actual pressures in our lives, but from our perceived lack of control over them. A study published in the *Journal of Hypertension* focused on the effects of stress in the workplace and, not surprisingly, found that people with excessive job-related stress invariably have hypertension. However, the most interesting finding in this study was that it is not the work itself but the lack of control people feel while at work that makes blood pressure rise. This might explain why more people suffer heart attacks at 9 A.M. on Monday mornings than at any other time of the week!

Marital strife, as Allison can attest, is also associated with hypertension. In a 1999 study published in the *American Journal of Hypertension,* Dr. Brian Baker and colleagues at the Toronto Hospital in Ontario, Canada, enlisted 134 men and 71 women with mildly elevated blood pressure who were not taking medications for hypertension. These men and women took standardized tests to measure their marital and job stress and were then hooked up to twenty-four-hour ambulatory blood pressure monitors, which measured their blood pressure around the clock, at home and at work. Among study subjects who were unhappy in their marriages, researchers found that the more contact they had with their spouse, the greater the likelihood of blood pressure increases. For these couples, more than four hours together caused a rise in blood pressure. On the other hand, the more time the happy couples spent together, the less likely they were to have elevations in blood pressure.

Whether your marriage is your hot button or there's something else in your life that is stressful to you, it is important that you be aware of the harmful effects unmanaged stress can cause. While you can't always avoid or change stressful situations, you can learn to modify your reaction to them.

▼ HYPERTENSION AND HIDDEN EMOTIONS

It is generally accepted that repressed emotions may result in depression, anxiety, and the like. Dr. Samuel J. Mann, of the Hypertension Center of the New York Hospital-Cornell Medical Center, makes a compelling case in his book *Healing Hypertension* that hypertension may be another consequence of hidden emotions. He contends that it is not the temporary elevations in blood pressure caused by responses to everyday stressors that contribute to hypertension. In fact, some studies demonstrate that people who express their anger tend to have lower blood pressure. Rather, it is the hidden emotions, the ones we aren't even aware we are harboring, that drive up blood pressure.

Hypertensive patients who fit this profile usually deny that they are under stress or that they have emotional problems. They may appear even more controlled and emotionally self-reliant than the average person. Yet they have a history of emotional stress, trauma, or unexpressed grief. Dr. Mann reports on patients with a longstanding history of hypertension who, after coming to terms with their emotions, experienced a return to normal blood pressure.

STRESS AND "PRE-HYPERTENSION"

As you may recall from Chapter 1, white-coat hypertension is the temporary rise in blood pressure caused by the anxiety of being in a medical setting and interacting with a health professional. The fear and anxiety aroused in this situation stimulate the sympathetic nervous system, which prompts a transient increase in blood pressure. While white-coat hypertension should not be confused with true hypertension, some experts warn that this phenomenon may represent an early stage in the development of true hypertension. Dr. M. A. Weber of the University of California claims that people who experience white-coat hypertension have virtually all of the metabolic and cardiovascular characteristics of hypertension. In comparing these individuals with patients who have been diagnosed as hypertensive, Dr. Weber notes similarities such as heightened norepinephrine and renin activity. He contends that people who are susceptible to white-coat hypertension are more likely to experience anxiety in other situations and are prone to the kind of chronic stress that leads to hypertension.

Among the most significant contributors to psychological stress is our fast-paced lifestyle. If you're working long hours, eating erratically, and feeling frustrated by heavy traffic and nonstop telephone calls, watch out! This is the kind of daily stress that contributes to the development of hypertension or exacerbates the condition if you already have it. Ineffective methods of "coping" with prolonged stress—drinking, smoking, overeating, and other unhealthy habits—may also induce or exacerbate hypertension.

TIPS ON HOW TO MANAGE STRESS

I don't advocate attempting to eliminate stress, because I am not convinced that it's possible. Sure, you can cut something out here or there to free up some time, or you can learn to avoid consistently stressful situations, but life is inherently stressful. My advice is, instead of struggling to eliminate stress—which only creates more stress—learn to manage it. With all of the evidence pointing to stress as a risk factor for all manner of illness, you can't afford not to.

I want to tell you about some simple techniques that will help alleviate your stress. As a bonus, these techniques will foster healthier blood pressure levels, lift your spirits, and enrich your daily life. By incorporating one or more of these stress-reducing tools into your daily routine, your psychological health will improve, and your physical health will surely follow.

De-stress with Sleep

One of the best stress busters is sleep. In our fast-paced lives, we give short shrift to sleep, but this activity, which takes up about a third of our entire lives, is critically important. Not only does your immune system shift into high gear while you are sleeping, but your brain takes the opportunity to wind down, sort out neural connections made during the previous day, and restore itself. Sleep deprivation has been linked with increases in infectious diseases and overall poor health, as well as declines in mood and mental function.

However, getting sufficient sleep may be especially important for people with hypertension. In a 1999 study published in the *American Journal of Hypertension*, Italian researchers explored the effects of sleep deprivation on 36 patients with high blood pressure. These patients, who had never been treated for hypertension, wore twenty-four-hour ambulatory blood pressure monitors on two separate days. On one of the days, they got a good night's sleep, while on the other they were allowed to sleep only from 3 A.M. to 7 A.M. It was discovered that during the night of inadequate sleep, the normal nighttime decreases in heart rate and blood pressure were diminished—and blood pressure was elevated the next morning, compared with readings after a good night's sleep. Furthermore, norepinephrine levels also increased during the night of interrupted sleep.

If you're among the estimated one in three Americans who sleep only six hours a night or less, you may be raising not only your stress levels but also your blood pressure. Although our sleep needs are individualized—it's not true that everyone needs eight hours a night—getting less than your body needs takes its toll. Yet sleep is often elusive, especially as we get older. Age-related declines in certain hormones and neurotransmitters contribute to poor sleep for the elderly.

Here are a few tips to ensure you'll get a good night's sleep. Cut out the caffeine. Although most of caffeine's effects are noted immediately after ingestion, it remains in the bloodstream for up to six hours. So that late-afternoon coffee break may be keeping you awake. One alcoholic drink before bed may help you fall asleep, but any more than that disrupts sleep patterns significantly. Light sources in your bedroom—even dim ones—may also disrupt sleep, as light interferes with the production of melatonin, the hormone that regulates our body clock. So turn off the TV and draw the shades before you go to bed.

I do not prescribe drugs to treat insomnia. Sure, they help you fall asleep, but they actually impair sleep cycles and daytime functioning over the long run. They are also highly addictive and have a host of negative side effects. Instead I recommend these tried-and-true natural remedies: melatonin, 5-hydroxytryptophan (5-HTP), valerian, and kava. Look for these safe, natural sleep aids in your health food store and use only as directed.

Ginseng: The Antistress Herb

Ginseng has been used in Asia for centuries to enhance stamina, reduce fatigue, and revitalize the body. However, research begun in the 1950s indicates that this herb's most powerful property may be its ability to modulate the harmful effects of stress. Ginseng belongs to an exclusive class of substances known as *adaptogens,* meaning they have diverse actions that help the body adapt to physical, mental, and biochemical stressors. The most popular type of ginseng is Korean ginseng (*Panax ginseng*). Phytochemicals called ginsenosides in *Panax ginseng* help balance the activities of the hypothalamus and the pituitary and adrenal glands, which are intimately involved in the stress response. This herb has been demonstrated to enhance performance during stressful mental and physical tasks, improve concentration, and decrease fatigue. A recent Mexican study showed that ginseng also offers overall benefits. In this double-blind study, people taking ginseng for four months reported noticeable improvements in quality of life, sense of well-being, mood, relationships, energy level, sexuality, and sleep.

Siberian ginseng (*Eleutherococcus senticosus*), a cousin of *Panax ginseng*, contains phytochemicals called eleutherosides that also have adaptogenic and stress-reducing properties. Siberian ginseng increases resistance to physical and psychological stress, fatigue, and illness and has also been demonstrated to improve the ability to tolerate heat, noise, and motion.

The recommended daily dose of *Panax ginseng* is 75 to 150 milligrams (standardized to contain 7 percent ginsenosides), and of Siberian ginseng 150 to 300 milligrams (standardized for 0.8 percent eleutherosides). Ginseng should be used cyclically—taken daily for two months, then off for at least two weeks. This cycle may be repeated as often as required. *Panax* and Siberian ginseng can be used alone or in combination with each other. Some experts warn that high doses of ginseng may cause insomnia, jitteriness, heart palpitations, and, in some people, elevated blood pressure. However, a thorough search of the medical literature does not support this claim. Although I would not recommend that you take ginseng without closely monitoring your blood pressure, I feel that if stress is a concern of yours, a trial of ginseng is warranted. Make sure you closely monitor your blood pressure the first two or three weeks of the trial period, never exceed the recommended dose, and take a break from it every two months, as suggested. If you observe an increase in your blood pressure while taking ginseng, discontinue it at once. If you are pregnant or nursing, consult a physician before using ginseng.

Calm Down with Kava

A common side effect of chronic stress is anxiety. Patients with anxiety are often given prescriptions for tranquilizers or other medications. I never prescribe these drugs, as they have a long list of side effects, including impaired concentration and memory, loss of coordination, sleep disturbances, and depression. Instead, I recommend that my patients take kava (*Piper methysticum*) for anxiety. The roots of this South Pacific plant contain kavalactones, which act in the deep recesses of the brain to produce feelings of calm and peacefulness. And rather than dulling the mind, kava actually improves concentration and memory. Furthermore, kava is extremely effective in reducing anxiety. In a 1991 study, 58 patients with symptoms of anxiety were divided into two groups. One group was given 100 milligrams of kava three times a day, while the other took a placebo. After four weeks the patients taking the herb had significant reductions in nervousness, heart palpitations, chest pains, dizziness, headaches, and gastrointestinal symptoms, compared with the placebo group.

For anxiety, consider giving kava a try. The suggested dose is 150 milligrams one to six times a day of an extract containing 30 percent kavalactones. Take no more than two capsules every four hours or six capsules in any twenty-four-hour period. Kava should be taken for a maximum of three months, then discontinued for two to four weeks before the cycle is repeated. Kava should not be taken before driving or operating heavy machinery, so it is best taken in the evening. Alcohol, tranquilizers, and other substances that affect the central nervous system should be avoided when taking kava.

The Power of Touch

Another great stress buster is touch. Your skin is your largest organ, and it needs care and attention. Touch brings your skin to life and has a profound effect on all of us—it lifts mood and enhances personal relationships. Did you know that newborns can actually die if they are deprived of touch? If you have a companion you love dearly, touch him or her. Hug. Hold hands. Link elbows. It's an incredible connection, and both of you will benefit from it. Likewise, extend a hand or open your arms to your acquaintances. You may be surprised how meaningful these simple gestures of greeting and affection can be for everyone involved.

Massage Therapy

Nothing quite parallels the relaxation and sense of being cared for as a massage. Massage is a useful and integral part of the healing process. It helps the body and spirit by improving blood and lymphatic flow and loosening tight muscles. With massage, you can experience the healing sensation of touch, while receiving the extra benefit of tension relief in tired, aching muscles. Most people wait until they're tied up in knots before they treat themselves to a massage. My suggestion is that you schedule appointments regularly. Many gifted massage therapists are available and trained in a variety of techniques. Call your local health club, consult the yellow pages, or see Appendix E to find a massage therapist in your area. If professional massages are out of the question, consider a "massage exchange" with a family member or friend—one week you get a massage, the next week you give one.

Pet Therapy

Pets nurture the body, mind, and soul, and if more doctors prescribed pets for hypertension, I'm convinced we'd see a rapid decline in blood pressure and heart disease. This is especially true for people who live alone and don't have the luxury of hugging or cuddling a loved one. The idea of pet therapy was first started by the Quakers at the York Retreat asylum in the eighteenth century. Today, pets are used in many medical settings, including half of all nursing homes throughout the country. Joseph S. Alpert, M.D., past chairman of the American Heart Association's Council of Cardiology, says, "Pets are tremendously important as companions for people with heart disease. The more restricted one's life is because of the disability, the more important the pet is."

Studies show that people with pets generally have lower blood pressure and heart rates than people without pets. Some of the most extensive research along these lines was performed in Australia at the Baker Medical Research Institute and the Alfred Hospital in Melbourne. Researcher Warwick P. Anderson, Ph.D., and colleagues did a three-year study of 5,741 men and women ages 20 to 60. They concluded that pet owners had lower blood pressure, triglycerides, and cholesterol levels than did nonowners. In the April 1996 *Medical Journal of Australia,* Dr. Anderson wrote, "Last year a comprehensive survey of pet ownership involving 1,011 interviews found that . . . pet owners were treated less frequently than non-owners for hypertension (8.6 percent vs. 12.9), hypercholesterolemia (2.3 vs. 3.5) or for 'a heart problem' (3.7 vs. 4.9)."

Pets are great reciprocators of touch. They beg to be petted, cuddled, and loved. In the process, they give all that back to you and more. Being greeted at the front door by Fritzi, my 13-year-old wirehaired terrier, and Lacy, our young Labrador retriever, when I come home is one of the small highlights of my day. A few minutes spent caressing or playing with your furry friend can lower stress as effectively as a glass of wine.

Deep Relaxation

Deep relaxation is the process of systematically relaxing your body and freeing your mind of busy thoughts. Sit or lie comfortably, preferably alone. Then begin to still your mind and reduce the busy thoughts that tend to dominate your consciousness. If you can't seem to quiet the rush of ideas, don't fight it. Just make a mental note of the thoughts you may want to return to later, and your mind will eventually grow still. Breathe naturally. Your daily commitment to this process will allow you to go deeper and deeper into relaxation. If you feel you need to focus your thoughts to help you relax, as many do, you might try the six-step relaxation exercise described in *The Relaxation Response,* by Herbert Benson, M.D., whom I mentioned earlier in this chapter. Dr. Benson developed this method to help people achieve deep relaxation. I've summarized the six steps for you here:

1. Sit or lie quietly in a comfortable position.
2. Close your eyes.
3. Deeply relax all of your muscles, concentrating on one after the other, beginning with your feet and progressing up your body to your face. Keep all of your muscles relaxed.
4. Breathe through your nose. Become aware of your breathing. As you breathe out, silently repeat the word "one" (or any other word of your choosing, such as "God" or "peace"). Breathe easily and naturally.
5. Continue this relaxing process for 10 to 20 minutes. You may open your eyes to check the time, but do not use an alarm clock. When you finish, remain reclined or seated quietly for a few minutes.
6. Don't worry about whether you are successful in achieving a deep level of relaxation. Maintain a neutral, passive attitude and allow relaxation to occur at its own pace. With practice, the desired response should come with little effort.

This practice is not as simple as it sounds. Some people find it easier to do with a guided relaxation tape. The one I use in my clinic to teach deep relaxation is called *Transforming Stress into Stillness,* by Dr. Vicki Weissler. The tape leads you through a deep relaxation session. Once you get the hang of it, the tape is optional. Many yoga classes offer instruction in deep relaxation as well. The important thing is to practice this technique regularly.

Deep Breathing Reverses Hypertension

Another powerful stress-reducing—and blood-pressure-lowering—tool to consider is deep breathing. Quick, shallow breathing can increase blood pressure by decreasing the kidneys' ability to excrete sodium. This effect was demonstrated in a 1995 study published in *Psychosomatic Medicine.* Researchers also found that deep breathing exercises may play an important role in the management of hypertension. Slow, deep, rhythmic breathing is the best way to regulate your breath and naturally bring your blood pressure down. Here is a simple deep breathing exercise you can perform anytime, anywhere:

1. Make yourself comfortable.
2. Begin breathing to this count: Inhale, two, three, four. Hold, two, three, four. Exhale, two, three, four. Hold, two, three, four.
3. Repeat the exercise two or three times.

You'll find this simple breathing exercise particularly helpful in calming yourself during stressful situations. If you find yourself getting worked up as you sit idly in heavy traffic or stand in a slow-moving line, try deep breathing. It helps to quickly relax your body and quiet your mind, and it just might lower your blood pressure.

Take a Music Break

Listening to music is another powerful stress reduction technique that reaches people emotionally and intellectually. It has been scientifically proven that certain types of music lift the mood, alleviate anxiety, and improve cognitive function. The type of music you choose depends on your individual taste, but to foster emotional peace and relaxation, I recommend flowing instrumental music. Some selections I personally like include "Air on the G String" by J. S. Bach, "Shepherd Moon" by Enya, or "Misty Mountain Melody" by Nature's Ensemble. However, any music you find relaxing is fine. Sit down, relax, and let your mind travel with the music. I also recommend playing soothing music in the background as you go about your chores. The next time you think about turning on the television set, turn on your ears instead and listen to music. This is much more relaxing than the constant blare of television, and besides, so much of what is on television these days is enough to raise anyone's blood pressure!

Smell Stress Away with Aromatherapy

Whenever you get a whiff of something, odor molecules are drawn to the millions of olfactory receptors high inside your nose and delivered directly to the brain. Smells are processed in the area of the brain associated with memories and emotions, which explains the strong emotional overlay of certain scents. They also activate the hypothalamus, which as you know governs basic involuntary functions, including the stress response. The use of specific scents for therapeutic purposes, *aromatherapy*, has undergone a resurgence of popularity in recent years. It has been scientifically proven that certain scents have dramatic effects on our physical and emotional state— they alter brain waves and actions of the sympathetic nervous system. One of the best studied is lavender, which has been demonstrated to have calming, relaxing, and sedative properties. This fragrance has been used as a replacement for sedative medications in nursing homes to relieve anxiety and facilitate sleep.

A few drops of lavender or another highly concentrated essential oil in a pot of simmering water or aroma diffuser fills your room with a refreshing, calming fragrance that just might lower your blood pressure. Here is a brief list of essential oils known to relieve stress and promote peace and calm.

- Basil°
- Bergamot
- Cardamom

- Cedarwood*
- Chamomile
- Geranium
- Jasmine
- Lavender
- Melissa (lemon balm)
- Rosemary*
- Sandalwood
- Ylang-ylang

*Not recommended for use during pregnancy.

Try These Soothing Teas

Certain herbal and tonic teas are recognized for their calming effects. Sipping a soothing cup of tea can be just the thing to help you unwind. So take a break, slow down, put the kettle on, prepare the tea, fill your cup with steaming water, and let the tea release its fragrance as it steeps. Smell it. Feel the heat. Take a sip. And let the world spin around for a few minutes without you. This is a good way to allow stress to slip from your body and mind.

Here are some choice teas to consider:

- *Chamomile.* It's the perfect tea just before bedtime, or for a relaxing midday break. Chamomile is an excellent nerve tonic and helps digestion.
- *Yerba mate.* This tonic tea from South America is known to strengthen the immune system, to defend against allergies, and to relieve constipation. Yerba mate is also somewhat energizing, yet it won't keep you awake the way caffeinated beverages do.
- *Peppermint.* This tea will soothe you while it stimulates your digestive system, relieving intestinal gas and ridding you of heartburn.
- *Oat straw.* This is one of the best teas for relaxing your nerves and taking the frazzle out of your day. It also does wonders for anyone trying to curb alcohol intake. Rumor has it that oat straw tea also has a mild aphrodisiac effect.

IN SUMMARY

Getting a handle on stress, anxiety, or depression can make a significant difference in your blood pressure and overall health. You must make a conscious, active choice to do something to minimize psychological stress. Consider some of these suggestions:

1. Use at least one of the techniques I've outlined for you in this chapter—or another of your choice—to combat stress. Choose the tools that seem most natural to you, and take a few minutes and give them a try. Regardless of the other stress-reducing techniques you use, make sure you also get a good night's sleep.
2. Create a relaxation routine in your life. For example, choose a certain time of the day—each and every day—to take time out just for yourself and do something you find relaxing.
3. Use a relaxation tool whenever you are feeling particularly stressed. In a situation where most people might reach for a drink or a cigarette, you could choose to listen to a relaxation tape or have a quiet cup of tea.
4. Remember that deep breathing exercises have been shown to help reduce blood pressure. Do the simple breathing exercise described earlier while you're stuck in traffic or standing in line for groceries, or anytime you're feeling especially stressed.

CHAPTER 15

Additional Therapies for Hypertension

"Prior to arriving at your door, I had a twenty-five-year history of hypertension and medication with prescription drugs. The result was that each year my blood pressure continued to go higher and the side effects of the largely unsuccessful drugs became greater and more unbearable. I was taking drugs to manage the side effects of other drugs to manage the side effects of those drugs. On medication, the usual reading of my blood pressure ranged from 180/96 at rest to 210/110 while moving. During the latter years I was having problems with chest pains and had to be careful while exercising.

"Because of unbearable side effects, one year before I entered your clinic I arbitrarily stopped taking all drugs. Within a very short time my blood pressure was 200/110 and frequently up to 240/130, especially during modest movement. I was duly warned that my chances of living an additional two years were at best 50 percent. This is when I started to look for alternative therapies.

"At the Whitaker Wellness Institute I have completed thirty hours of EECP [Enhanced External Counterpulsation], and today while I was completing my twenty-fifth hour of chelation, my blood pressure was 145/82. This is still a bit high, but I did not get my problem in a short time and I certainly do not expect to solve it overnight. I no longer have any chest pains, even while exercising. The changes in lifestyle, in diet, and in exercise have given me a chance to enjoy my senior years with a bit of vigor and happiness. I do not know whether it was the EECP or the chelation or the prescribed diet with vitamins *and minerals, but I now consider myself in very good health, and I give full credit for this to the treatment I received there."*

We have covered in detail the essential Whitaker Wellness program for preventing and reversing hypertension: nutritional supplementation, diet, water, exercise, and stress reduction. However, as a medical doctor I have had the opportunity over the years to test the merits of other promising therapies that must be administered by a medical professional in a clinical setting. Three therapies have stood the test of time, and I have incorporated them into my medical practice. They have benefited hundreds of patients at my clinic, such as the patient who wrote the above letter, with conditions ranging from atherosclerosis and angina to diabetic circulatory complications and hypertension.

You will probably not find these therapies at your conventional doctor's office—they have not gained a foothold among conventional physicians. Why this is I cannot explain. These therapies are effective: clinical trials demonstrating their benefits have been published in peer-review medical journals. They are safe and have none of the side effects of the drugs that kill over 100,000 Americans and hospitalize a million more every year. And compared with the astronomical costs of long-term medication usage, hospitalization, and surgical treatment for undiagnosed or poorly treated hypertension and atherosclerosis, they are relatively inexpensive. Although I believe that most of you will be able to effectively lower your blood pressure by the methods previously discussed in this book, I want you all to be aware of these powerful therapies and discuss them with your doctor.

EECP DRAMATICALLY IMPROVES CIRCULATION

Enhanced External Counterpulsation (EECP) was first developed by Harry Soroff, M.D., at Harvard University more than forty-five years ago. EECP is a noninvasive therapy used primarily in the treatment of poor circulation and angina pectoris (chest pain associated with heart disease). But it is also an up-and-coming therapy for hypertension. EECP lowers blood pressure by dramatically improving circulation, thereby decreasing resistance on the "pipes." It was also shown to increase the release of nitric oxide, which relaxes, dilates, and widens the arteries to further contribute to lower blood pressure. It increases blood flow by pumping—actually squeezing—blood from the lower extremities. While you lie flat or at a slight angle on a table, what looks like thick panty hose or a wet suit is wrapped around your lower extremities from your ankles to just below your waist. Then, in time with the beat of your heart, it contracts, forcing blood through the extremities and increasing its flow through the arteries of your heart, trunk, and upper body. The improved circulation to these areas also brings valuable oxygen and nutrients where they are needed most. It has long been known that as arteries become clogged, the heart will open up additional avenues of blood around the blockages, called *collateral circulation*. With EECP, the counterpulsation of the blood flow rapidly increases the development of collateral circulation and restores blood flow. A treatment session lasts about an hour, and aside from the squeezing sensation, there is no discomfort or danger whatsoever. A usual course is 35 one-hour treatments, given once or twice daily. In just three to seven weeks—far less time than it takes to recuperate from bypass surgery—tremendous improvements are noted.

In a 1992 study published in the *American Journal of Cardiology*, 18 patients with chronic angina who had already had surgery and were being treated with medication were given five EECP treatments a week. After the full course, 16 of the 18 patients reported complete relief of angina, while the other 2 had some improvement. Thallium stress tests showed 100 percent resolution of the obstructive flow in 12 of the patients, partial reduction in 2, and no change in 4. In another study, 12 patients initially reported an average of 3.9 episodes of chest pain per day, at a pain rating of 2.9 on a scale of 1 to 4 (with 4 being the most painful). After a full course of EECP, the pain episodes were reduced to an average of 0.1 per day (one episode every ten days) with an intensity of only 1.7. All patients reported improvements in their energy levels, ability to work, and overall sense of well-being.

I found out about EECP from one of my own patients, B.D., who was initially scheduled to have bypass surgery more than eight years ago. Following a strict diet and exercise program and undergoing chelation therapy, he did extremely well with no symptoms and no need for drugs whatsoever for five years. About three years ago, possibly because he's a hard-driving, type-A businessman, B.D.'s chest pain came back with a vengeance. He researched therapies around the world, found EECP, and asked me to evaluate it, which I did. B.D. underwent a course of thirty-five treatments and experienced dramatic improvements in his angina and his overall quality of life. Whereas he once needed to take nitroglycerin regularly, he is now almost completely drug-free and performs exercises he was formerly unable to do without experiencing severe pain.

Although most of the U.S. research on EECP has been done on angina, EECP has been used in China for decades for the treatment of many conditions that involve poor circulation—hypertension, erectile dysfunction, diabetic eye problems, intermittent claudication, and kidney disease, to name a few. I highly recommend this therapy for patients with atherosclerosis and hypertension, especially patients who do not respond to other therapies. Despite the fact that EECP was developed at one of the most prestigious medical centers in this country and has been used abroad for decades, until recently it was ignored in the United States. In the past year, however, the viability of this therapy has finally been recognized by insurance companies and even by Medicare. The primary reason for their interest is economics. A course of EECP costs a fraction of that of bypass surgery—and the likelihood of complications that add more to costs is minuscule. Unfortunately, you may be hard pressed to get your insurance company or Medicare to reimburse for EECP for anything except angina that is not amenable to surgery. That doesn't mean it will not help with hypertension or the other conditions previously discussed.

This remarkable therapy deserves easier and broader accessibility. As its merits become more obvious in future years—and I have no doubt they will—EECP may become a standard tool in the treatment of hypertension. To locate a facility where EECP is administered, see Appendix E.

REVERSE ATHEROSCLEROSIS WITH EDTA CHELATION THERAPY

EDTA chelation (pronounced *key-LAY-shun*) is a procedure used to remove accumulated minerals and heavy metals from the body. The name chelation is appropriate, as the Greek origin of the word, *chele,* means claw, and EDTA chelation grabs on to minerals and expels them from the body. Chelation involves the intravenous administration of a manmade amino acid called ethylene diamine tetraacetic acid (EDTA). Once in the bloodstream, EDTA latches on to heavy metal ions, forming a tight chemical bond with them. As EDTA passes through the kidneys, it is expelled from the body, taking with it toxic heavy metals and excess iron, copper, and calcium. By removing these unwanted minerals, EDTA chelation helps to loosen and remove arterial plaque, thereby restoring the artery wall to a healthier state. This helps reduce high blood pressure by improving blood flow and reducing resistance on arteries and arterioles.

EDTA chelation first gained popularity in the 1940s, when it was used to treat victims of toxic metal poisoning. Men employed in painting World War II battleships with lead-based paint often suffered the ill effects of acute lead poisoning, and EDTA was the most efficient way of removing it from the body. It was discovered in a serendipitous manner that these men receiving chelation therapy for heavy metal poisoning had remarkable improvements in chest pain and leg discomfort due to impaired circulation associated with atherosclerosis. Enthusiasm grew for this effective, noninvasive therapy for heart and vascular disorders, and clinical results were overwhelmingly positive.

However, over the next few years, as drugs and surgical procedures for the treatment of cardiovascular disease gained popularity, chelation fell out of favor. This is yet another example of a valuable therapy's being rejected not on scientific grounds or as a result of negative controlled clinical trials, but by the bias of conventional medicine. Despite its well-documented safety and efficacy, EDTA chelation therapy has been the subject of unfounded negative publicity. Nevertheless, a few hundred physicians have continued to offer the therapy, and over the years almost a million satisfied patients have received EDTA chelation with often remarkable results.

How much research is behind EDTA? According to Garry F. Gordon, M.D., D.O., an expert on chelation therapy, "There are 7,000 known articles in our possession about EDTA, and I am sure if I hired somebody and we really went to work, there would be another 3,000 that we haven't found. This would amount to about 10,000 articles on EDTA." Dr. Gordon also points out that chelation has a long and strong safety record. When administered properly by a physician, intravenous EDTA has an extremely low risk of side effects. It is substantially less dangerous than bypass surgery and is one of the best therapies I know of to prevent premature death from heart attack or stroke.

I do want to address a couple of the safety concerns raised about EDTA chelation therapy. One is that since EDTA is a nonspecific mineral chelator, it might remove certain essential minerals from the body. Zinc, for example, is easily chelated, so EDTA could, in theory, induce a zinc deficiency. The same is true of calcium, magnesium, and potassium, which, as you recall, are important for healthy blood pressure. To counter the possibility of deficiencies in important minerals, physicians often add magnesium and other minerals to the IV bottle, and patients are encouraged to take a high-dose multivitamin and mineral supplement such as that recommended in Chapter 10. Another concern is that since chelation removes calcium from the body, it might have an adverse effect on bone density, a valid concern for those suffering from or at risk for osteoporosis. However, it has been demonstrated that as EDTA removes calcium from the bloodstream and the arteries and washes it out through the kidneys, through a complex activity involving the parathyroid gland it simultaneously *stimulates* bone growth.

Chelation is administered in a doctor's office. A chelation session typically lasts about three hours, and patients undergo sessions one to three times per week for a total course of twenty to thirty treatments. Except for the initial IV needle insertion, the procedure involves little, if any, discomfort, and in my thirteen years of utilizing chelation therapy, I have observed very few complications or side effects. I recommend EDTA chelation therapy for patients with hypertension, atherosclerosis, angina, and circulatory conditions such as intermittent claudication and diabetic complications of the lower extremities. For information on how to locate a physician in your area who administers chelation, contact the American College for Advancement in Medicine (see Appendix E).

LOWER BLOOD PRESSURE THE ANCIENT CHINESE WAY

Acupuncture is an ancient Chinese healing art with a 5,000-year history. It is based on the concept of Qi (pronounced *chee*), the life energy that permeates all living things. Qi flows through the body in a dozen channels called meridians. More than 400 specific sites along these meridians, known as acupuncture points, connect with specific areas of the body. When Qi is blocked by stress, poor diet, fatigue, or other disturbances, disease results. Acupuncture simply unblocks the flow of Qi to restore energy flow and balance the body.

Although acupuncture is most often used to treat pain conditions such as headaches and arthritis, it has been demonstrated to effectively improve a number of conditions, including hypertension. Exactly how acupuncture lowers blood pressure has been explored in many studies. It is felt to reduce the secretion of several hormones and other messenger chemicals involved in blood pressure control, including renin (the enzyme produced in the kidneys that sets the RAAS into motion) and aldosterone (the hormone that causes sodium and water retention). In a 1997 study carried out in Taiwan, 50 patients with hypertension not taking antihypertensive drugs were treated with acupuncture. When their blood pressures taken thirty minutes after treatment were compared with pretreatment measurements, decreases were observed in both systolic blood pressure (from 169 to 151 mm Hg) and diastolic blood pressure (from 107 to 96 mm Hg). Decreases were also noted in renin secretion.

Acupuncture involves the insertion of hair-thin, sterilized, disposable needles in the acupuncture points where Qi is blocked. Amazingly, this doesn't hurt, although you might feel a tingling or mild aching sensation when the needles are twisted to "grab the Qi." The

needles remain inserted for ten to thirty minutes, during which time
you rest. Many report a profound sense of peace and relaxation during acupuncture treatments. Some conditions require only one or two
treatments, but most chronic problems require several sessions.
Acupuncture is extremely safe, and side benefits—versus side effects
of drugs—often occur. It has been observed, for example, in studies
of acupuncture's effects on blood pressure, that levels of blood lipids
often fall and heart rhythms normalize.

If your blood pressure does not respond to the therapies outlined
in this program for reversing hypertension—or if you want another
tool in your quest for normal blood pressure—I suggest you give
acupuncture a try. To locate a licensed acupuncturist in your area,
refer to Appendix E.

IN SUMMARY

If your blood pressure remains elevated in spite of following the
lifestyle and supplement recommendations in this program for reversing hypertension, consider one of these therapies:

1. Enhanced External Counterpulsation (EECP).
2. EDTA chelation therapy.
3. Acupuncture.

CHAPTER 16

Get Started Now!

Joan had a long history of hypertension—she had been on blood pressure medications for forty of her sixty-two years. She also had a strong family history of hypertension and had resigned herself to a life of medication. Over the years, however, Joan had developed an interest in alternative medicine, and the more she learned, the more convinced she became that there had to be a better way. She read about the Whitaker Wellness Institute's weeklong Back to Health program in my newsletter, Health & Healing, *and she and her husband decided to give it a try.*

Her first day at the clinic was devoted to intensive testing and evaluation, including an exercise stress test and an echocardiogram. During her initial consultation her blood pressure was slightly high at 144/84, even though she was taking a beta-blocker drug. Under the close supervision of her physician she was advised to cut her drug dosage in half while starting on a comprehensive nutritional supplement program consisting of high doses of antioxidants, B-complex vitamins, essential fatty acids, magnesium and other minerals, garlic, and hawthorn.

Joan and her husband enjoyed their week at the clinic. They stayed at the first-class, full-service hotel where our program takes place, and dined with the other patients on heart-healthy gourmet meals prepared by our chef. They participated in daily exercise classes led by our physical therapist and attended lectures by the physicians and professional staff on diet, exercise, stress reduction, nutritional supplementation, and alternative approaches to common conditions.

They enjoyed getting to know the other patients, several of whom had similar health challenges. Joan had a consultation with our certified nutritionist, who worked up a personalized meal plan for her. Every day Joan's blood pressure was monitored, and it held steady, even though she was taking only half the medication she had previously taken.

She saw her doctor again later in the week for reevaluation and was surprised at the strides she had made in only a few days. Her blood pressure had remained in good control all week, so her doctor recommended that she gradually discontinue her medication altogether. Joan left the clinic energized and motivated to stick with the program—and she did. When I spoke to her eight months later she had lost 20 pounds, her blood pressure was maintained in the 120/70 range, and for the first time in years she felt in control of her health.

Joan is typical of the patients who go through the Back to Health program at the Whitaker Wellness Institute. Her response, after living, eating, and breathing an optimal lifestyle for a week, was, "Hey, I can do this!" The improvement she experienced in one short week was a powerful motivator, as was the support of the others facing similar health challenges.

I have some patients who swear that one particular component of the program is what did it for them. They latched exclusively onto the diet, for example, and felt that it alone made the difference. Or they started exercising, which was enough in itself to normalize their blood pressure. However, for the vast majority of individuals with hypertension, no single aspect of this multistep program can be given all the credit. It is the *combination* of diet, supplementation, exercise, increased water intake, and stress reduction that is the ticket.

The human body responds beautifully when it is given the proper tools it needs to heal itself. That is why a disciplined approach to the nutritional and lifestyle guidelines discussed in this book can restore normal blood pressure. Your only side effects on this program will be a slimmer, trimmer physique; lower cholesterol and triglyceride levels; better blood sugar control; a healthier cardiovascular system; and more energy than you ever dreamed of. Even if you have a family history of hypertension or have been on high blood pressure medication for years, you can succeed with this approach. It is my sincere desire to help you get your blood pressure into the healthy zone as soon as possible.

Conventional western medicine cannot cure what it does not understand. Chronic diseases and conditions such as hypertension, heart disease, and diabetes are primarily conditions of lifestyle. That is a fact, and it is why no single factor will remedy your hypertension—but the right combination will. So let's bring it all together into a program you can live with. This is the same program I recommend for my patients with hypertension at the Whitaker Wellness Institute, and the majority of them are able to bring their blood pressure under control.

▼ POTENTIAL SIDE BENEFITS OF THIS PROGRAM

- Improved sense of energy and well-being
- Weight loss
- Lower cholesterol and triglyceride levels
- Better blood sugar control
- Increased circulation
- More sexual vitality
- Improved immunity
- Better memory and cognitive function
- Decreased risk of stroke, heart attack, and diabetes
- Increased life span

To make it even easier for you to put the pieces together, in this chapter I have recapped my key recommendations from the earlier chapters. Look them over and see how they fit together in one sensible, natural approach for reducing your blood pressure. By implementing these important lifestyle changes, you will be well on your way to a healthier, happier life.

WORK WITH YOUR PHYSICIAN

If you are taking any medications for high blood pressure, be sure to work with your physician to gradually reduce your dosages as you begin to implement the natural therapies recommended in this book. NEVER quit any medication on your own—always consult your physician first. You can monitor your own progress by taking blood pressure readings at home, which will give you and your doctor an extra edge in determining which therapies work best for you. (See Appendix D for detailed instructions on measuring your own blood pressure.)

GET NUTRITION INSURANCE WITH NUTRITIONAL SUPPLEMENTS

Boost your nutrient intake with a broad-spectrum multivitamin and mineral supplement and/or single-nutrient supplements. The best time to take supplements is with meals, as they are best absorbed when your gastrointestinal system is geared up to digest food. Also be sure to divide your daily supplements between two or three meals. Here is a recap of the nutrients I recommend for hypertension, and the daily dose of each:

Antioxidants:	Vitamin C	2,500 milligrams
	Vitamin A	5,000 international units
	Beta-carotene	15,000 international units
	Vitamin E	800 international units
B vitamins:	Folic acid	800 micrograms
	Vitamin B-6	75 milligrams
	Vitamin B-12	100 micrograms
Minerals:	Magnesium	1,000 milligrams
	Calcium	1,000 milligrams
	Potassium	99 milligrams
	Chromium	200 micrograms
	Vanadyl sulfate	45 milligrams
	Selenium	200 micrograms
	Zinc	30 milligrams

Essential fatty acids:	Fish oil capsules	2,000 milligrams
Herbs:	Garlic	Supplemental equivalent of 1 to 2 cloves
	Hawthorn	360 milligrams of an extract standardized for 1.8 to 2.2 percent vitexin flavonoids
Miscellaneous:	Coenzyme Q10	180 to 200 milligrams
Amino acids:	Arginine*	1–2 grams 3 times a day

*For best absorption, avoid eating protein at the same time you take arginine; carbohydrates are okay.

BALANCE YOUR MINERALS

Bring your sodium-potassium levels into balance by stepping up your potassium intake and reducing your salt consumption. Remember this important ratio: consume at least four times as much potassium as you do sodium. Do this by eating potassium-rich plant foods, and using a potassium-based salt substitute such as Nu-Salt. Also eat magnesium- and calcium-rich foods, per the lists in Chapter 9, and take enough supplemental magnesium to total an average of 1,000 milligrams per day, balanced with an equal amount of supplemental calcium.

REDUCE YOUR BODY FAT

Obesity is the number one factor related to hypertension. In some cases, shedding excess fat alone returns blood pressure to normal levels. As I explained on page 39, a body mass index (BMI) of 19 to 25 is in the healthy range; 26 and above puts you at increased risk for hypertension, syndrome X, and other degenerative diseases. There are three basic ways to reduce your body fat: eat less fat, eliminate sugar and refined carbohydrates, and exercise regularly. You can accomplish your goal by sticking to the Whitaker Wellness Diet for High Blood Pressure outlined in Chapter 11 and by adhering to a regular exercise program such as the one described in Chapter 13. If you follow these recommendations, weight loss will come naturally, allowing you to achieve your ideal weight and reduce your blood pressure.

STOP THESE UNHEALTHY HABITS

Smoking is a major contributor to hypertension. When you stop smoking, you will not only reduce your blood pressure, you will also dramatically decrease your chances of a heart attack. Studies have shown that ten years after quitting, the heart attack risk of a former pack-a-day smoker is roughly the same as that of a nonsmoker. Make a commitment now and fill out the contract on page 46. It will be one of the best things you do in your quest for lower blood pressure and overall improved health.

Alcohol in moderate doses—one to two drinks a day—appears to have some health advantages, but the dangers of exceeding this amount are very well documented. If you are on the Quick Start Diet, I want you to avoid alcohol completely. Once you begin the Whitaker Wellness Diet for High Blood Pressure, one or at most two drinks per day is acceptable. However, do not *start* drinking in an effort to improve your health.

EAT (LOW-GLYCEMIC), DRINK (WATER), AND BE HEALTHY

If you have severe stage 3 hypertension (systolic pressure of 180 mm Hg or higher, or diastolic pressure of 110 mm Hg or higher) follow the Quick Start Diet for one to six weeks (see Chapter 11 for details). Once your blood pressure is out of the danger zone, start with and stick to the Whitaker Wellness Diet for High Blood Pressure. This program addresses all of the known dietary factors involved in hypertension and insulin resistance. Try the menu suggestions and recipes (Appendix C) to make this portion of the program delicious and easy.

Hydrate your body by drinking plenty of water—aim for ten to twelve 8-ounce glasses of water per day. Remember to build up to this amount slowly, and consult with your doctor if you have kidney disease or congestive heart disease. Make sure the water you drink has been purified, and drink extra water when you exercise—one or two glasses before you exercise and after you finish. If your workout is particularly long or strenuous, rehydrate every 10 to 15 minutes with 4 to 6 ounces of water.

EXERCISE YOUR BODY, MIND, AND SPIRIT

Make regular physical exercise a part of your life. Choose a form of exercise you enjoy and stick to it on a consistent basis. I recommend that you get a minimum of 30 minutes of low- to moderate-intensity exercise four to five times per week. A walking program, such as the one described in Chapter 13, works well for many people. Use the exercise log on page 188 to help you commit to and accomplish your exercise goals. Consider exercising with a friend, which will help keep you on track and make your regimen more social and fun.

Reduce stress. Although you can't completely eliminate stress from your life, you can learn to manage it. The tools I advocate are medicinal herbs, ginseng and kava; adequate sleep; therapeutic touch, massage, and reflexology; deep relaxation, deep breathing, music, aromatherapy, and soothing teas. Make stress management a daily ritual—carve out some time each day to quiet your mind and relax your body.

TRY EECP, CHELATION THERAPY, AND/OR ACUPUNCTURE

Enhanced External Counterpulsation (EECP), EDTA chelation therapy, and acupuncture are excellent adjuncts to this basic program for reversing hypertension. EECP dramatically improves circulation and facilitates the creation of collateral circulation. EDTA chelation cleans up your arteries, which allows blood to flow more freely and blood pressure to come down. Acupuncture also lowers blood pressure, most likely by affecting levels of hormones involved in blood pressure regulation.

CONGRATULATIONS ON YOUR COMMITMENT TO OPTIMAL HEALTH

By implementing the steps in this comprehensive program, you are well on your way to reversing hypertension. I am convinced that as you follow the guidelines outlined in this book, you will agree that the best treatment for hypertension is a natural therapeutic approach supported by a healthy lifestyle. Always remember that natural therapies are not an overnight cure. This program may require some time for your body to adjust to, so be patient. I applaud your willingness to take charge of your health and make changes in your life. The rewards are well worth your efforts, for you will be adding quality years to your life.

APPENDIX A

ANTIHYPERTENSIVE DRUGS

Thiazide Diuretics

Aquatensen and Enduron (methyclothiazide)
Diuril, Mykrox, and Zaroxolyn (metolazone)
Diuril (chlorothiazide)
Hydrodiuril, Microzide, and Oretic (hydrochlorothiazide)
Hygroton and Thalitone (chlorthalidone)
Lozol (indapamide)
Naturetin (bendroflumethiazide)

Potassium-Sparing Diuretics

Aldactone (spironolactone)
Dyrenium (triamterene)
Midamor (amiloride)

Loop Diuretics

Bumex (bumetanide)
Demadex (torsemide)
Edecrin (ethacrynic acid)
Lasix (furosemide)

Beta-Blockers

Blocadren (timolol)
Cartrol (carteolol)
Coreg (carvedilol)
Corgard (nadolol)

Inderal and Inderal LA (propranolol)
Kerlone (betaxolol)
Levatol (penbutolol)
Lopressor and Toprol (metoprolol)
Normodyne and Trandate (labetalol)
Sectral (acebutolol)
Tenormin (atenolol)
Zebeta (bisoprolol)

ACE Inhibitors

Accupril (quinapril)
Altace (ramipril)
Capoten (captopril)
Lotensin (benazepril)
Mavik (trandolapril)
Monopril (fosinopril)
Prinivil and Zestril (lisinopril)
Univasc (moexipril)
Vasotec (enalapril)

Long-Acting Calcium Channel Blockers
Adalat CC, Procardia XL (nifedipine)
Calan SR, Covera HS, Isoptin SR, and Verelan (verapamil)
Cardene SR (nicardipine)
Cardizem, Dilacor XR, and Tiazac (diltiazem)
DynaCirc, DynaCirc CR (isradipine)
Norvasc (amlodipine)
Plendil (felodipine)

Central Adrenergic Inhibitors

Aldomet (methyldopa)
Catapres (clonidine)
Hylorel (guanadrel)
Ismelin (guanethidine)
Serpasil (reserpine)

Tenex (guanfacine)
Wytensin (guanabenz)

Angiotensin II Receptor Blockers

Avapro (irbesartan)
Cozaar (losartan potassium)
Diovan (valsartan)

Combination Drugs

Beta-blocker—diuretic
  Corzide (nadolol with bendroflumethiazide)
  Inderide (propranolol with hydrochlorothiazide)
  Lopressor HCT (metoprolol with hydrochlorothiazide)
  Tenoretic (atenolol with chlorthalidone)
  Timolide (timolol with hydrochlorothiazide)
  Ziac (bisoprolol with hydrochlorothiazide)
ACE inhibitor—diuretic
  Capozide (captopril with hydrochlorothiazide)
  Lotensin HCT (benazepril with hydrochlorothiazide)
  Prinzide, Zestoretic (lisinopril with hydrochlorothiazide)
  Vaseretic (enalapril with hydrochlorothiazide)
Angiotensin antagonist with diuretic
  Hyzaar (losartan with hydrochlorothiazide)
ACE inhibitor—calcium channel blocker
  Lexxel (enalapril with felodipine)
  Lotrel (benazepril with amlodipine)
  Tarka (trandolapril with verapamil)
  Teczem (enalapril with diltiazem)
Others
  Combipres (clonidine with chlorthalidone)
  Minizide (prazosin with polythiazide)

APPENDIX B

KEEPING TRACK OF YOUR BLOOD PRESSURE

Week	1	2	3	4	5	6	7	8	9	10	11	12
Blood Pressure (systolic/diastolic)												
Weight												
Exercise (number of workouts per week)												
Diet (rate on a scale of 1 to 5 with 1 being in line with recommendations in this program and 5 being "out of control")												
Water (average number of glasses per day)												
Stress Management (number of times relaxation tools used)												

Figure 11. Weekly Blood Pressure Chart

APPENDIX C

THE WHITAKER WELLNESS DIET FOR HIGH BLOOD PRESSURE

TWO-WEEK MENU PLAN

(*Indicates that recipes are included here.)

WEEK 1

Monday

Breakfast
*Fruit salad with yogurt and nuts
*Cinnamon toast

Lunch
*Vegetable soup
*Spinach-mushroom salad with fat-free Italian dressing
Whole wheat crackers
Orange

Dinner
Mixed spring greens with olive oil and balsamic vinegar dressing
*Vegetable lasagna
Garlic bread (sprouted-grain bread, toasted then lightly drizzled
    with olive oil and rubbed with a clove of cut garlic)
*Strawberries with yogurt sauce

Tuesday

Breakfast
Hot oatmeal with blueberries and chopped walnuts, skim milk, rice
  milk, or soy milk
Half grapefruit

Lunch
*Asparagus and leek tart
Broccoli, tomato, and red onion salad served with nonfat ranch dressing
Rye crackers
Apple

Dinner
*Cucumber salad
*Grilled chicken with couscous and mushroom teriyaki sauce
Fresh green beans
*Poached fruit

Wednesday

Breakfast
*French toast made with sprouted whole-grain bread
*Poached apples sweetened with stevia and cinnamon
Nonfat cottage cheese

Lunch
Boca Burgers (soy)* on whole-grain sprouted bun with lettuce,
  tomato, red onion, and sprouts
Green salad with *flaxseed oil dressing
Melon slice

Dinner
*Miso soup with tofu and green onions
Vegetable stir-fry served over buckwheat noodles
Mixed berries

*Boca Burgers and other soy-based burgers are available in the frozen foods section of
health food stores and some supermarkets.

Thursday

Breakfast
Multigrain hot cereal with skim milk, rice milk, or soy milk
Sliced peaches

Lunch
*Winter bean soup
*Greek salad with olive oil and balsamic vinegar dressing
Sprouted-grain toast
Tangerine

Dinner
Spinach-mushroom salad
*Grilled salmon with yogurt-dill sauce
*Curry-spiced couscous
Yellow squash, snow peas, and red peppers
*Spiced pears

Friday

Breakfast
*Egg white scramble
Sprouted whole-grain bagel with nonfat cream cheese
Grapefruit

Lunch
*Vegetarian chili
*Oriental coleslaw
Whole wheat crackers
Plums

Dinner
Mixed greens with olive oil and balsamic vinegar
Spaghetti with turkey *marinara sauce
Sprouted-grain garlic bread
*Berries with yogurt sauce

Saturday

Breakfast
Oatmeal with blueberries and chopped walnuts, skim milk, rice
    milk, or soy milk
Sprouted-grain toast

Lunch
*Tostada
Pear slices

Dinner
*Pasta primavera
Lettuce and tomato salad with *flaxseed oil dressing
*Apple crisp

Sunday

Breakfast
*Veggie omelet
Sprouted-grain toast
Apricot slices

Lunch
*Chef's salad
Sprouted-grain bagel with nonfat cream cheese
Melon slice

Dinner
Broiled or sautéed chicken breast
Baked sweet potato
Green beans
Spinach salad
*Berry crisp

WEEK 2

Monday

Breakfast
Hot multigrain cereal with skim milk, rice milk, or soy milk
Raspberries or blueberries

Lunch
*High-potassium soup
Tossed green salad with olive oil and balsamic vinegar dressing
Sprouted-grain bread
Apple

Dinner
*Garlic-and-peppers shrimp
*Couscous pilaf
Sautéed yellow squash and zucchini
*Spiced pear

Tuesday

Breakfast
*Spicy oat pancakes with unsweetened applesauce and cinnamon
Nonfat yogurt
Fresh strawberries

Lunch
*Chef's salad
100% whole-grain rye bread
Orange

Dinner
*Spinach-tofu sauté
Snow peas sautéed with water chestnuts
Brown rice
Fresh raspberries garnished with mint

Wednesday

Breakfast
Buckwheat kasha with skim milk, rice milk, or soy milk
Plain nonfat yogurt
Plums

Lunch
*Garlic gazpacho
*Spinach-mushroom salad with fat-free Italian dressing
Whole wheat crackers
Tangerine

Dinner
*Ginger-yogurt chicken
Steamed broccoli and cauliflower
*Cucumber salad
Sprouted-wheat bread
Blackberries with *yogurt sauce

Thursday

Breakfast
*Fruit salad with yogurt and nuts
Sprouted-grain bagel with nonfat cream cheese

Lunch
*High-energy salad with lemon–olive oil dressing
100% whole-grain rye bread
Orange

Dinner
*Tofu steaks
Cooked barley
Steamed yellow squash and cauliflower
Pumpernickel bread (made with 100% rye flour)
*Spiced pear

Friday

Breakfast
*Veggie omelet
Toasted sprouted whole-grain bread
Peach slices

Lunch
*Mulligatawny soup
Cucumber-tomato salad with *flaxseed oil dressing
Sprouted whole-grain pita bread
*Green garlic dip (used as spread for pita bread)

Dinner
Mixed spring greens with olive oil and balsamic vinegar
Baked cod with fresh dill
*Couscous
Mandarin orange slices (packed in water)

Saturday

Breakfast
Oatmeal with skim milk, rice milk, or soy milk
Chopped apples and walnuts

Lunch
*Tabouli
*Vegetable soup
Rye crackers
Applesauce

Dinner
Chicken grilled with rosemary
Brown rice
*Oriental coleslaw
Fresh cherries

Sunday

Breakfast
♦French toast
Fresh peaches
Yogurt

Lunch
Tuna sandwich (oil-free) on whole wheat pita bread
Green salad

Dinner
♦Asparagus chicken
Brown rice
Mixed baby greens salad with olive oil dressing
Steamed broccoli and summer squash
♦Apple crisp

RECIPES

These recipes were put together with the assistance of the Whitaker Wellness Institute chef, Idel Kelly, and nutritionist, Diana Lara, M.S.

BREAKFAST DISHES

Fruit Salad with Yogurt and Nuts
   1 apple, cored and cut into chunks
   1 pear, cored and cut into chunks
   ½ cup fresh berries
   2 tablespoons *each* raw almonds, sunflower seeds, and pumpkin
      seeds
   6 tablespoons plain nonfat yogurt
Mix fruit, nuts, and seeds. Stir in yogurt.
Serves 2.

Cinnamon Toast
   2 slices sprouted-grain bread
   2 teaspoons brown rice syrup
   ½ teaspoon cinnamon
Brown one side of bread under broiler. Turn, spread on syrup and sprinkle with cinnamon, then brown this side under broiler for a minute or so.
Serves 2.

Egg White Scramble
   ½ bell pepper, chopped
   ½ onion, chopped

6 egg whites
3 tablespoons skim milk
¼ cup nonfat cottage cheese (optional)
Olive oil cooking spray
Nonfat sour cream

Brown peppers and onions in skillet, adding a little water as needed; set aside. In a bowl, scramble egg whites with skim milk and cottage cheese. Pour onto heated, nonstick skillet coated with olive oil cooking spray. Cook gently, turning with spatula as needed, till done to taste. Stir in vegetables. Serve with a dollop of nonfat sour cream.
Serves 2.

French Toast

4 egg whites or 2 egg whites and one whole egg
4 tablespoons skim milk, rice milk, or soy milk
½ teaspoon vanilla
½ teaspoon cinnamon
2 slices sprouted whole-grain bread
Olive oil cooking spray
Topping of choice

Mix egg whites, skim milk, vanilla, and cinnamon. Dip bread in egg mixture. Cook on a nonstick griddle sprayed with olive oil cooking spray, turning bread slices until brown on both sides. Serve with fruit-juice-sweetened jams, unsweetened applesauce, or poached fruit (recipe in dessert section).
Serves 2.

Spicy Oat Pancakes

1 cup skim milk or soy milk
1 tablespoon white vinegar
1 cup old-fashioned rolled oats
¼ cup soy flour
¼ cup rice flour
¼ teaspoon cinnamon
2 egg whites, beaten
Olive oil cooking spray
Sliced fresh fruit

Mix skim milk with vinegar and let stand for about 10 minutes. Combine the dry ingredients separately. Blend the milk mixture with egg whites and stir into the dry ingredients. Let the batter stand for about 2 hours, allowing it to thicken. Spoon batter onto skillet with olive oil cooking spray. Turn pancakes just once and remove from skillet when golden brown. Serve topped with sliced fresh fruit.
Serves 2 or 3.

Veggie Omelet

¼ cup *each* chopped mushrooms and onions
Olive oil cooking spray
2 egg whites and 1 whole egg
2 teaspoons water

Sauté vegetables in water. Mix eggs with water and beat lightly. Heat nonstick pan over medium heat, coat bottom with cooking spray, and pour in eggs. Shake pan gently and lift edges of omelet as eggs cook, tilting pan to let uncooked eggs run underneath. Slide finished omelet from pan, top with vegetables, and fold in half.
Makes 1 omelet.

SOUPS

Vegetable Soup

3 cloves garlic, chopped
¼ cup chopped fresh basil (optional)
¼ cup chopped parsley
½ cup chopped celery
½ cup chopped onion
6 cups low-sodium, nonfat chicken or vegetable broth
1 cup water
1 can (28 oz.) whole tomatoes, no-salt, chopped
1 zucchini, sliced
1 summer squash, sliced

1 head broccoli, cut into small pieces
Ground black pepper to taste

In a large, nonstick stockpot, cook the garlic, basil, parsley, celery, and onion for about 3 minutes, stirring to brown evenly and adding water by the tablespoon, as needed. Add broth, water, and tomatoes. Bring to a gentle boil. Add remaining vegetables and simmer on medium heat for 20 to 30 minutes, or until vegetables are tender. Add pepper to taste. (You may substitute any of your favorite vegetables in this recipe. One cup of beans also make a nice addition.)

Serves 6.

Miso Soup with Tofu and Green Onion

2 cups low-sodium, nonfat chicken or vegetable broth
¼ cup cubed firm tofu
2 tablespoons miso (found in Asian markets or health food stores)
1 tablespoon chopped green onion

Heat broth and tofu in a saucepan until hot. Mix miso with 2 tablespoons water to thin, then add to broth and mix well, just before serving. Garnish with chopped green onion.

Serves 2.

Winter Bean Soup

2 cups low-sodium, nonfat chicken or vegetable broth
1 can (28 oz.) whole tomatoes, mashed
1 medium turnip, chopped small
¼ teaspoon dried red pepper (optional)
½ teaspoon ground black pepper
1 leek, sliced (white part only)
½ bunch Swiss chard, chopped small (green part only)
¼ yellow onion, chopped
1 clove garlic, chopped
1 can (16 oz.) cannellini or white kidney beans
½ cup cooked barley

In a large stockpot, place broth, mashed tomatoes, turnip, dried red

pepper, and black pepper. Bring to a boil. Reduce heat and simmer for 20 to 25 minutes. In another pan, place leek, Swiss chard, onion, and garlic, adding water as needed. Sauté for 3 to 4 minutes, until soft. Add to stockpot and simmer for another 20 minutes, then add beans and barley. Cook for 10 minutes.
Serves 6.

Vegetarian Chili

  3 cans (28 oz. each) whole tomatoes, no-salt
  4 cups cooked pinto beans
  ½ cup onion, chopped
  ½ cup bell pepper, chopped
  2 teaspoons chili powder, or to taste

Mix all ingredients, mashing whole tomatoes before adding to mixture. On low heat, simmer for 1 hour, adding water as needed.
Serves 6.

High-Potassium Soup/Broth

You may use this recipe as a substitute (broth only) for recipes requiring low-sodium, nonfat broth. Or you can serve it as a vegetable soup (see details below).

  10 celery stalks
   2 leafy greens (beet tops, collards, turnip greens, kale, etc.)
   2 sweet potatoes, peeled
   2 onions
   3 cloves garlic
   1 pound summer squash
   1 pound zucchini
   2 bunches parsley

Wash and chop vegetables, place in an 8-quart pot, and cover with water. Bring to a boil and then turn heat down to a simmer. Simmer for 30 minutes, turn off heat, and allow to sit (covered) for another 30 minutes. For broth: remove the vegetables and discard them (the nutrients remain in the broth). For soup: simply heat and serve. The soup keeps for about a week in the refrigerator.
Serves 6.

Garlic Gazpacho

4 cloves garlic
1 cucumber, peeled
1 pound tomatoes
½ green pepper
1 cup low-sodium, nonfat chicken or vegetable broth
4 ounces sodium-free spicy tomato juice
1 tablespoon olive oil
¼ cup chopped fresh cilantro
½ teaspoon ground white pepper
2 tablespoons chopped green onions
Extra cilantro for garnish

Peel and mince the garlic. Coarsely chop cucumber, tomatoes, and green pepper, and combine with garlic in a large bowl. Add broth, tomato juice, and olive oil. Toss lightly and top with green onions and cilantro for garnish. Add pepper. Chill the soup for at least 2 hours before serving.
Serves 4.

Mulligatawny Soup

½ cup chopped onion
½ cup chopped celery
½ cup chopped green pepper
½ cup chopped turnip
½ cup chopped apple
Dash crushed red pepper
¾ teaspoon curry powder
1 tablespoon olive oil
3 cups low-sodium, nonfat chicken or vegetable broth
1 teaspoon arrowroot or cornstarch, mixed with 3 tablespoons water
¾ cup garbanzo beans (pureed in blender)
1 cup diced, cooked chicken (optional)
Chopped parsley (for garnish)

Sauté vegetables, apple, red pepper, and curry powder in olive oil over low to medium heat until tender. Set aside. Heat stock in a

saucepan to boiling point. Add arrowroot or cornstarch mixture and stir constantly until it returns to a boil. Add sautéed vegetables, pureed beans, and chicken (optional). Heat to serving temperature. Garnish with chopped parsley.
Serves 4.

SALADS

Spinach-Mushroom Salad
1 bunch spinach, cleaned and stemmed
4 ounces mushrooms, sliced
2 hard-boiled egg whites, chopped
1 small Bermuda onion, chopped
Fat-free Italian dressing

Combine first 4 ingredients and serve with dressing.
Serves 4.

Cucumber Salad
1 cucumber, peeled and thinly sliced
½ cup rice vinegar
½ teaspoon coarsely chopped fresh ginger
½ teaspoon lightly toasted sesame seeds

Combine cucumber, vinegar, and ginger. Chill for 2 hours. Remove ginger before serving. Garnish with sesame seeds.
Serves 2.

Flaxseed Oil Salad Dressing
3 tablespoons fresh, unprocessed flaxseed oil
2 tablespoons balsamic vinegar (or lemon juice)
1 small clove garlic, pressed
Dash ground black pepper
Dash chopped parsley
Dash sodium-free seasoning

Blend all ingredients together and serve immediately. Olive oil may be substituted for flaxseed oil.
Serves 2.

Greek Salad

¼ pound gourmet salad mixture
3 cucumbers, peeled and sliced
½ red onion, thinly sliced
3 tomatoes, chopped
1 cup artichoke hearts packed in water, drained
¼ cup fresh basil, chopped
1 cup fat-free Italian dressing
1 tablespoon crumbled feta cheese

Combine all ingredients. Let marinate in refrigerator for at least 2 hours.
Serves 6.

Oriental Coleslaw

Dressing
¼ cup low-sodium soy sauce
½ cup sesame oil
2 tablespoons rice vinegar
2 tablespoons Dijon mustard
½ teaspoon grated fresh ginger
1 teaspoon brown rice syrup

Salad
1 medium head cabbage
2 carrots
1 small can mandarin oranges
2 to 3 tablespoons toasted sesame seeds

Blend dressing ingredients together. Shred cabbage and carrots and place in large bowl. Fold dressing into cabbage-carrot mixture. Discard juice from mandarin oranges. Spoon orange segments over coleslaw and top with toasted sesame seeds.
Serves 12.

Chef's Salad

⅔ cup chopped romaine lettuce, rinsed and drained
⅔ cup chopped fresh spinach, rinsed and drained
½ cup kidney beans, rinsed and drained
2 cups chopped raw vegetables (celery, broccoli, cauliflower, cucumber, green peppers, radishes, tomatoes, mushrooms, onions) in bite-sized pieces, rinsed and drained
2 ounces skinless turkey breast, cut in strips
2 ounces low-fat Swiss cheese, cut in strips
Fat-free salad dressing

In a large mixing bowl, toss together the lettuce and spinach. Add the kidney beans and the chopped vegetables. Top with turkey and Swiss cheese strips. Pour dressing over salad and toss well.
Serves 2.

High-Energy Salad

4 cups gourmet salad mix
1 ripe avocado, cubed
½ cup sliced fresh mushrooms
½ cup chopped red cabbage
2 celery stalks, sliced
½ cup grated zucchini
8 large radishes, sliced
1 cup alfalfa sprouts
4 tablespoons minced cilantro

Toss all vegetables, except radishes, sprouts, and cilantro—use these to garnish salad. Serve with lemon–olive oil dressing (below).
Serves 4.

Lemon–Olive Oil Dressing

2 tablespoons freshly squeezed lemon juice
3 tablespoons olive oil
1 clove garlic, crushed
Freshly ground black pepper, to taste
Sodium-free seasoning, to taste

Blend all ingredients.
Serves 2.

Green Garlic Dip

  2 cloves garlic, chopped
  1 large ripe avocado
  6 ounces soft tofu
  3 tablespoons fresh lemon juice
  ⅛ teaspoon cayenne pepper

Add all of the ingredients to a blender or food processor and blend until creamy. Use for dipping fresh vegetables or as a spread for crackers.

Serves 2.

Tabouli

  2 cups boiling water
  1 cup bulgur
  2 tablespoons olive oil
  2 tablespoons fresh lemon juice
  3 tablespoons finely chopped fresh mint
  ½ teaspoon dulse or Nu-Salt
  ¼ teaspoon ground black pepper
  2 large tomatoes, diced
  ½ cup chopped onion

Pour boiling water over the bulgur, stir, and let stand for 1 hour. Drain bulgur in a fine-meshed strainer or cheesecloth, discard the water, and press out excess water with the back of a slotted spoon. Fluff the bulgur with a fork. Mix the olive oil, lemon juice, mint, dulse or Nu-Salt, and pepper in a separate medium-sized bowl, adding tomatoes, onion, and drained bulgur. Let the salad mixture chill in the refrigerator for several hours.

Serves 4.

MAIN DISHES

Marinara Sauce

This sauce can be used in the lasagna recipe or over any type of pasta.

    1 cup sliced mushrooms

    1 green pepper, chopped

    1 onion, chopped

    2 cans (28 oz.) whole tomatoes, chopped

    3 cloves garlic, minced

    Pinch of oregano

    ½ cup chopped flat-leaf parsley, or to taste

    ¼ cup chopped fresh basil, or to taste

Mix all ingredients in a saucepan and simmer.

Makes about 8 cups.

Vegetable Lasagna

    1 zucchini, finely chopped

    1 yellow squash, finely chopped

    1 carrot, finely chopped

    4 cups fat-free ricotta cheese

    ¼ teaspoon nutmeg

    2 26-ounce jars low-fat, low-sodium spaghetti sauce (or recipe above)

    1 pound lasagna noodles, cooked according to package directions

Mix vegetables with ricotta cheese and nutmeg. Cover until ready to use. In a 9 x 13-inch rectangular baking dish, add a layer of sauce, followed by a layer of cooked noodles, then a layer of ricotta-vegetable mixture. Repeat with 2 more layers of sauce, noodles, and ricotta, and end with an extra layer of sauce. Cover and bake at 350 degrees for approximately 1 hour. Top with sauce before serving.

Serves 8.

Asparagus and Leek Tart

½ pound asparagus spears, trimmed and cut into 2-inch pieces
2 leeks, sliced (white part only)
2 tablespoons flour
8 egg whites, lightly beaten
1 cup nonfat ricotta cheese
¼ cup shredded low-fat, low-sodium Swiss cheese
½ cup skim milk
¼ teaspoon nutmeg
2 teaspoons olive oil
½ cup crumbled 100% whole-grain sprouted-wheat bread

Preheat oven to 425 degrees. Boil 3 inches water in a large pan. Blanch asparagus for 2 to 3 minutes. Drain and set aside. In a medium pan, sauté leeks over medium heat for 4 to 5 minutes, sprinkle in flour, stir to coat, and transfer mixture to a large bowl. Add eggs, ricotta cheese, Swiss cheese, milk, and nutmeg, and mix again. Meanwhile, add olive oil to bread crumbs, pat flat into bottom of a pie pan, and toast in the oven for 5 to 6 minutes, or until browned. Cool for 10 minutes. Pour egg-cheese mixture over browned bread crumbs. Bake until puffy and brown, about 40 minutes. Let stand 10 minutes before slicing.
Serves 6.

Grilled Chicken with Couscous and Mushroom Teriyaki Sauce

2 boneless chicken breasts, 4 to 6 ounces each
⅛ cup light soy sauce
¾ cup water
1 tablespoon apple juice concentrate
½ teaspoon rice vinegar
2 cups sliced mushrooms
1 clove garlic, or to taste, minced
1 cup cooked couscous (see below)

Grill chicken breasts. Meanwhile, in a saucepan combine soy sauce, water, apple juice concentrate, vinegar, mushrooms, and garlic. Simmer about 15 minutes. Pour over chicken and couscous.
Serves 2.

Couscous

Couscous consists of small grains of pasta and is a staple of North African cuisine. It cooks very rapidly and can be flavored with the following (per cup of *uncooked* couscous):

Curry couscous—add ½ to 1 teaspoon curry powder along with water

Couscous pilaf—add up to ½ cup cooked, finely chopped onion, sliced mushrooms, chopped green pepper, peas, etc.

Oriental couscous—add 1 teaspoon low-sodium soy sauce along with water

Tostadas

   2 whole wheat tortillas
   1 cup cooked, mashed pinto beans
   1 cup shredded lettuce, romaine preferred
   1 tomato, chopped
   2 green onions, chopped, or ¼ cup chopped onion
   ¼ cup grated low-fat cheese
   Salsa

Heat tortillas in a nonstick skillet (no oil required). Heat the beans in a saucepan. Spread half the beans on each tortilla and top with remaining ingredients.
Serves 2.

Grilled Salmon with Yogurt-Dill Sauce

   2 salmon fillets, 4 ounces each
   ½ cup plain nonfat yogurt
   ½ teaspoon chopped fresh dill (or ¼ teaspoon dried dill)

Grill salmon for about 5 minutes on both sides. Put grilled fish into a baking dish, cover, and bake in oven for 10 to 15 minutes to replace moisture. Combine yogurt and dill and serve on top of salmon.
Serves 2.

Pasta Primavera

½ pound fresh broccoli florets, cut into bite-sized pieces
½ pound zucchini, cut into thin diagonal slices
½ pound fresh mushrooms, sliced thin
Olive oil cooking spray
1 cup ripe tomatoes, chopped
1 pound firm or extra-firm tofu, in small cubes
2 cloves garlic, minced
½ cup chopped parsley
Ground black pepper to taste
1 pound linguini noodles
1 tablespoon olive oil
1 to 2 tablespoons water
2 tablespoons grated Parmesan cheese

Steam broccoli florets over boiling water until crisp-tender. Set aside. Rinse and drain zucchini and mushrooms. In a large skillet coated with olive oil cooking spray, lightly sauté garlic. Add a small amount of water while sautéing, if necessary. Add the zucchini and mushrooms. Cook, covered, over low heat for 5 minutes. Add the steamed broccoli, tomatoes, parsley, and pepper. Mix well and cook 2 minutes longer. Cook the linguini in a large pot of boiling water according to package directions. When done al dente, drain well and return to the pot. Stir in olive oil and 1 to 2 tablespoons of water. Add the vegetables and grated Parmesan cheese. Toss well and serve hot.

Serves 8.

Garlic-and-Pepper Shrimp

5 cloves garlic (or less, if this scares you)
1 green pepper
1 yellow pepper
1 red pepper
2 tablespoons olive oil
1 tablespoon low-sodium soy sauce
2 tablespoons water

20 large shrimp, peeled and deveined
Cooked brown rice to serve 4

Peel garlic and slice cloves lengthwise. Seed peppers and cut them into ½-inch strips. Heat oil in a large pan and sauté the peppers and garlic for 1 minute. Add shrimp and stir-fry until they turn bright pink. Serve over brown rice.
Serves 4.

Spinach-Tofu Sauté

1 tablespoon olive oil
¼ cup sliced green onions
½ pound firm tofu, cubed
¼ cup pitted black olives
1 tablespoon minced fresh dill (or ½ tablespoon dried dill)
3 tablespoons vegetable broth
1 pound fresh spinach, cleaned and stemmed

Heat olive oil in a large skillet and lightly sauté green onions. Add tofu, olives, dill, and vegetable broth. After 1 minute of gentle stirring, add the spinach to the mixture and continue stirring for 1 more minute.
Serves 4.

Ginger-Yogurt Chicken

2 chicken breast halves, 4 to 6 ounces each
1 teaspoon olive oil
1 cup nonfat yogurt
¼ cup toasted whole wheat or sprouted-grain bread crumbs
1 teaspoon freshly grated ginger, or ground ginger to taste

Brown the chicken on both sides in the olive oil. Mix the yogurt, bread crumbs, and ginger. Arrange chicken in a single layer in an oven-safe dish and spread yogurt mixture over the surface of each piece of chicken. Bake uncovered in a 325-degree oven for 30 minutes, or until chicken is done.
Serves 2.

Tofu Steaks

1 pound extra-firm or firm tofu
2 teaspoons low-sodium soy sauce
Olive oil cooking spray

Firm tofu has a high water content, so to remove some of the water before cooking, place the block of tofu on a plate and invert another plate on top of it. Fill a kettle or saucepan halfway with water to provide some weight, then carefully balance it on the top plate. Leave for 15 minutes or so, then drain off the water that has been pressed from the tofu. This makes it firmer so it won't fall apart while cooking. (With extra-firm tofu you can skip this step.) Slice tofu lengthwise into four slices. Sprinkle with soy sauce. Heat a skillet over medium to medium-high heat, spray with olive oil cooking spray, and sauté tofu for 3 to 5 minutes on each side.
Serves 4.

Asparagus Chicken

1 medium onion, chopped
2 cloves garlic, minced
1 tablespoon olive oil
3 cups asparagus spears, cut in one-inch pieces
1 cup sliced mushrooms
1 pound skinless, boneless chicken breasts, sliced into 2-inch
   strips
1 lemon, juice and grated peel
¾ cup low-sodium, low-fat chicken or vegetable broth
Freshly ground black pepper
3 tablespoons chopped parsley

Sauté onion and garlic in oil for about 3 minutes. Add asparagus and mushrooms and sauté for 3 more minutes. Remove from pan and set aside. Add chicken to the pan and sauté until lightly browned (about 3 minutes). Return the vegetables to the pan and add the lemon peel and juice, broth, and pepper. Stir mixture, allowing it to simmer for about 10 minutes. Add chopped parsley, stir, and remove from heat.
Serves 4.

DESSERTS

Berries with Yogurt Sauce

    2 cups of your favorite berries, whole or sliced

    2 teaspoons brown rice syrup

    ½ cup nonfat plain yogurt

Mash ⅓ cup berries with brown rice syrup. Mix in yogurt. Drizzle over remaining berries.

Serves 2.

Poached Fruit

    Water

    2 to 4 fresh apples, pears, peaches, or nectarines, cored or pitted and sliced

    ⅛ to ¼ teaspoon stevia or ¼ cup brown rice syrup or to taste

    ¼ teaspoon cinnamon (optional)

Put 1 inch of water in a saucepan. Add chopped fruit, stevia or syrup, and cinnamon (optional) and simmer for 5 to 10 minutes, just until tender. The fruit can also be mixed with plain yogurt or spooned over hot cereal or French toast.

Serves 2.

Apple Crisp

    2 cups apples, cut into small chunks

    ¼ cup water

    ¼ cup whole wheat flour

    ½ cup uncooked rolled oats

    2 teaspoons cinnamon

    ¼ cup chopped walnuts

    2 teaspoons walnut or olive oil

    2 tablespoons brown rice syrup

Spread the apples over the bottom of an 8 x 8-inch baking dish. Pour water over fruit. Combine flour, rolled oats, cinnamon, walnuts, and oil and mix well. Sprinkle this mixture over fruit. Drizzle with brown rice syrup. Bake at 350 degrees for 30 to 40 minutes, or until top is lightly browned.

Serves 8.

Spiced Pears

    1 firm pear, cored and halved
    ¼ cup brown rice syrup
    Pinch cinnamon
    2 tablespoons chopped, toasted almonds

Cover the bottom of a saucepan with 1 inch of water. Add pear halves, cover, and simmer over low heat for 5 minutes. Remove from pan with a slotted spoon. Add brown rice syrup, almonds, and cinnamon to pan and simmer over low heat for 5 minutes. Spoon sauce over pears.

Serves 2.

SNACKS

Raw sunflower and pumpkin seeds.

Raw almonds.

Raw vegetables.

Protein drink with soy powder.

Apples and raw almond butter.

Hummus dip with vegetables or crackers.

Tofu dips with vegetables.

100% rye crackers with raw almond butter.

100% rye crackers with avocado.

Fruit

½ sandwich: chicken, avocado, almond butter with brown rice syrup, or egg salad, tuna salad (use sprouted breads and mustard, nonfat yogurt, or mayo).

1 slice sprouted-grain bread with brown rice syrup and raw almond butter or tahini.

Herbal iced tea sweetened with stevia or xylitol (in place of soda and juice).

Nonfat cottage cheese or plain yogurt with fruit and natural sweeteners.

Raw soybeans in the pod (found in freezer section).

APPENDIX D

HOW TO MONITOR YOUR BLOOD PRESSURE WITH A SPHYGMOMANOMETER

Blood pressure self-monitoring is easy, accurate, economical, and more convenient than physician-administered exams. Blood pressure tends to be lowest upon waking, then rises somewhat as activities begin, with spikes possibly after meals, coffee breaks, or stressful events. Try to take your pressure at the same time(s) each day. The traditional approach to measuring blood pressure uses a sphygmomanometer, or an inflatable arm cuff and a stethoscope. Readings will vary based on body position—standing, sitting, or lying down—so be consistent. Here are the steps to monitoring blood pressure with a sphygmomanometer.

1. Pick a quiet spot.
2. Wrap the cuff around one arm just above your elbow.
3. Sit with the cuff-wrapped arm on a flat surface at "heart height."
4. Place the detachable blood pressure gauge on the table facing you.
5. Close the air-exhaust valve.
6. Locate your brachial-artery pulse on the little-finger side of your elbow crease.
7. Place the stethoscope under the cuff so that the sensor diaphragm rests on this pulse point.
8. Place the stethoscope earpieces in your ears.
9. Relax and breathe normally.

10. Inflate the cuff about 30 points (mm Hg) to about 200, or slightly higher. Adequate inflation produces a tourniquet effect, so you should hear no sound through the stethoscope.

11. Open the air valve gradually, so that the cuff deflates at about 3 mm Hg per second. This step may take practice. Quicker deflation produces inaccurate readings. The cuff continues to act as a tourniquet as long as the pressure inside it is greater than the pressure in the brachial artery. As soon as the cuff pressure drops below the arterial pressure, the pulse returns.

12. Keep your eyes on the gauge and listen for the first tapping pulse sound. The moment it becomes audible, the reading on the gauge indicates your systolic reading—the first, or top, number of the blood pressure fraction.

13. Continue releasing air and listening. As the tourniquet effect decreases, the pulse will become faint as unimpeded blood flow returns. When it disappears, the gauge reading indicates your diastolic pressure—the second, or bottom, number in the blood pressure fraction.

14. Open the air exhaust valve, release all air from the cuff, and remove it.

15. Wait two minutes or so and then repeat the process.

In addition to the classic blood pressure arm cuff, various high-tech computerized monitors are now available. Regardless of the technology running the blood pressure monitors, all work on the same principles. High-tech models just do more of the work for you. Computerized blood pressure monitors incorporate the stethoscope into the arm cuff to produce readings automatically. You simply turn the monitor on, wrap the cuff around your brachial artery, and wait for the reading to appear.

Work with your physician to achieve the best results from a self-monitoring program. Take your home monitoring device with you to an appointment and make sure you are using it correctly and that its readings are similar to those of the equipment in the doctor's office. Be sure to seek medical attention if your readings are abnormally elevated.

APPENDIX E

RESOURCES

Dr. Whitaker's Medical Clinic

Whitaker Wellness Institute
4321 Birch Street
Newport Beach, CA 92660
800-488-1550
www.whitakerwellness.com

Dr. Whitaker's medical clinic specializes in one-week programs that include:

- One-week residential program
- M.D. consultations
- Comprehensive medical testing
- Seminars on the latest in medical research and nutritional supplementation
- Personalized exercise programs
- Nutritional consultations
- Stress management instruction
- Individualized nutritional supplementation
- Specific therapies for various health conditions, including hypertension, heart disease, and diabetes
- Second opinion evaluations

ALTERNATIVE MEDICINE ORGANIZATIONS

American College for Advancement in Medicine
P.O. Box 3427
Laguna Hills, CA 92654
800-532-3688
www.acam.org
Send a self-addressed, stamped envelope with 55 cents postage to receive a listing of alternative health physicians—many of whom administer chelation therapy—and a listing of books and other resources available for purchase.

American Preventive Medical Association
459 Walker Road
Great Falls, VA 22066
800-230-2762
A political action group that offers a directory of practitioners, books, and other resources on alternative medicine.

COMPOUNDING PHARMACIES

For the location of compounding pharmacies in your area, contact the following:

International Academy of Compounding Pharmacies (IACP)
P.O. Box 1365
Sugar Land, TX 77487
800-927-4227
www.iacprx.org

Professional Compounding Centers of America (PCCA)
9901 South Wilcrest
Houston, TX 77099
800-331-2498
www.thecompounders.com

HEALTH INFORMATION

Dr. Whitaker writes a monthly newsletter, *Health & Healing*, covering breakthroughs in alternative medicine and offering safe solutions for our most common health concerns. For subscription information, contact:

Health & Healing
Phillips Publishing, Inc.
7811 Montrose Road
Potomac, MD 20854
800-539-8219
www.drwhitaker.com

INFORMATION ON SPECIFIC THERAPIES

Enhanced External Counterpulsation (EECP)
Vasomedical, Inc.
180 Linden Avenue
Westbury, NY 11590
800-455-3327
www.vasomedical.com
Provides information on EECP and a list of clinics offering this therapy.

Glycemic Research Institute
601 Pennsylvania Avenue N.W., Suite 900
Washington, DC 20004
Provides information on the glycemic index of foods.

National Certification Commission for Acupuncture and Oriental Medicine
11 Canal Center Plaza, Suite 300
Alexandria, VA 33214
703-548-9004
www.nccaom.org
Provides referrals to licensed acupuncturists.

PRODUCTS

Nutritional Supplements
Healthy Directions, Inc.
7811 Montrose Road
Potomac, MD 20854
800-722-8008, ext. 1638
www.healthydirections.com

Relaxation Tape
Transforming Stress into Stillness, Dr. Vicki Weissler
800-826-1500

Sulfonil (for Smoking Cessation)
Sound Nutrition
800-844-6645

Sun-Pure Water Purifier
Phillips Products & Services
800-705-5559, ext. 109

RECOMMENDED READING

Batmanghelidj, F. *Your Body's Many Cries for Water.* Global Health Solutions, Falls Church, VA, 1995.

Benson, Herbert. *The Relaxation Response.* Outlet Books, New York, 1993.

Burton Goldberg Group. *Alternative Medicine: The Definitive Guide.* Future Medicine Publishing, Puyallup, WA, 1993.

Eliot, Robert S. *From Stress to Strength: How to Lighten Your Load and Save Your Life.* Bantam Books, New York, 1994.

Fried, Robert and Merrell, Woodson C. *The Arginine Solution.* Warner Books, New York, 1999.

Moore, Richard D. *The High Blood Pressure Solution: Natural Prevention and Cure with the K Factor.* Healing Arts Press, Rochester, VT, 1993.

Murray, Michael. *Encyclopedia of Nutritional Supplements*. Prima Publishing, Rocklin, CA, 1996.

———. *The Healing Power of Herbs*. Prima Publishing, Rocklin, CA, 1995.

———. *Heart Disease and High Blood Pressure*. Prima Publishing, Rocklin, CA, 1997.

Murray, Michael and Pizzorno, Joseph. *Encyclopedia of Natural Medicine*. Prima Publishing, Rocklin, CA, 1998.

Whitaker, Julian M. *Is Heart Surgery Necessary?* Regnery Publishing, Washington, DC, 1995.

———. *Reversing Diabetes*. Warner Books, New York, 1987.

———. *Reversing Heart Disease*. Warner Books, New York, 1985.

Glossary

Abnormal glucose tolerance. The inability to properly metabolize blood sugar.

Aldosterone. A hormone that increases the amount of sodium and water in the bloodstream and raises blood pressure.

Ambulatory blood pressure monitoring test (ABPM). A twenty-four-hour test that accounts for the natural blood pressure fluctuations that occur throughout the day. Measures blood pressure at twenty- to thirty-minute intervals.

Aneurysm. A ballooning of the wall of an artery, vein, or the heart resulting from weakening of the wall by hypertension, injury, or disease. This condition is sometimes an abnormality present at birth.

Angiogram. The X-ray picture taken during an angiography. The chambers of the heart and/or blood vessels can be seen by using the specially injected contrast-medium, or dye.

Angiography. An X-ray examination of the chambers of the heart or blood vessels that is accomplished with a special fluid called a contrast-medium, or dye, which is visible by X ray. As fluid makes its way through the bloodstream, the X ray follows its course and makes pictures called angiograms.

Angiotensin-converting enzyme (ACE). An enzyme that reacts with angiotensin I to form angiotensin II, which contributes to hypertension.

Angiotensin-converting enzyme (ACE) inhibitors. A type of commonly prescribed antihypertensive medication that lowers blood pressure by blocking the enzyme that initiates the potent renin-angiotensin-aldosterone system (see below).

Angiotensin I. Produced by the interaction of renin and angiotensinogen under conditions of stress; converted to angiotensin II through the action of angiotensin-converting enzyme (ACE).

Angiotensin II. Produced by the enzymatic action of ACE upon angiotensin I. Causes the muscles of the arteries and arterioles to contract and the adrenals to release stress hormones; together, these drive up blood pressure.

Angiotensinogen. A protein produced in the liver on a continuous basis that interacts with the enzyme renin to form angiotensin I, which initiates the renin-angiotensin-aldosterone system (see below).

Antioxidant. Molecule capable of preventing damage to tissues by free radicals. Common antioxidants include vitamins C, E, A, and beta-carotene and the mineral selenium.

Aorta. The large artery that receives blood from the heart's left ventricle and delivers it for distribution throughout the body.

Aortic valve. A valve in the heart, located between the aorta and the left ventricle, which has three flaps that control the blood flow.

Apoplexy. See **Stroke.**

Arrhythmia. An abnormal rhythm of the heart, sometimes termed *dysrhythmia.*

Arterioles. Small branches of arteries with muscular characteristics. When arterioles contract, the blood flow is temporarily decreased, causing the pressure in the arteries (blood pressure) to increase.

Arteriosclerosis. Damage to and subsequent hardening of the major arteries. Free radicals and LDL cholesterol are primary causes of arterial damage and loss of elasticity.

Artery. Blood vessels that carry blood from the heart to the various parts of the body. Arteries have thick, elastic walls that can expand as blood flows through them.

Atherosclerosis. Buildup of fatty plaque in the artery walls. The layered, irregular buildup of plaque causes narrowing of the interior walls of the arteries. As a result, blood flow is increasingly reduced. Term used interchangeably with *arteriosclerosis.*

Atrium. Either of the upper two chambers of the heart, where blood collects before passing to the ventricles.

Baroreceptors. Specialized receptors in the aorta and arteries of the neck and thorax that send messages to the brain when modifications need to be made in blood pressure.

Beta-blockers. The second most widely prescribed type of antihypertensive medication (after diuretics). They lower blood pressure by blocking the heart's ability to respond to epinephrine and adrenaline.

Blood clot. A jellylike mass of tissue made of blood. It forms to stop the flow of blood after an injury. Blood clots can form inside arteries, resulting in an interruption of blood flow and thus a heart attack or stroke.

Blood pressure. The force exerted by blood as the heart pumps it through the arteries.

Blood vessels. The network of tubes, or "pipes," through which the blood circulates, including arteries, arterioles, veins, venules, and capillaries.

Body mass index (BMI). A standardized measurement of fat-versus-lean body composition.

Bradycardia. A slow heartbeat (less than 50 beats per minute).

Calcium channel blockers. A type of commonly prescribed antihypertensive medication that reduces blood pressure by preventing excess calcium from entering the cells, thus relaxing and dilating the arteries.

Capillaries. Microscopically small blood vessels between arteries and veins that end in branchlike capillary beds, where nutrients, gases, hormones, and other vital components are delivered to the tissues, and waste products of cellular metabolism are picked up.

Cardiac. Pertaining to the heart.

Cardiology. The study of the heart, its functions, and its condition in health and disease.

Cardiovascular disease (CVD). Any affliction of the heart or blood vessels.

Cardiovascular system. The circulatory system of the heart and blood vessels.

Carotid artery. The major artery in either side of the neck.

Cholesterol. A fatty substance that is found in all animal cells and that is an integral part of all membranes, as well as the precursor to the steroidal hormones. There are two major types of cholesterol, LDL cholesterol (which is deposited into artery walls) and beneficial HDL cholesterol (which ushers cholesterol out of the body). Dietary cholesterol is found only in animal foods, including whole-milk dairy products, meat, fish, poultry, animal fats, and egg yolks.

Coenzyme Q10. A naturally occurring substance involved in cellular energy production. CoQ10 is used therapeutically in the treatment of congestive heart failure, hypertension, and other cardiovascular diseases. Also known as *ubiquinone*.

Congestive heart failure (CHF). The inability of the heart to pump out all the blood that returns to it, resulting in a backup of blood in the veins that lead to the heart, and sometimes an accumulation of fluid in various parts of the body.

Coronary arteries. Two arteries arising from the aorta that arch down over the top of the heart, then branch and provide blood to the heart muscle.

Coronary artery disease. Narrowing of the coronary arteries so that blood flow to the heart is reduced. Also called *coronary heart disease*.

Diabetes. Disease in which the body is either deficient in insulin or fails to use insulin properly. Also referred to as *diabetes mellitus*.

Diastolic blood pressure. The blood pressure that occurs when the heart muscle is relaxed between beats. This is the second, or bottom, number in a blood pressure reading such as 120/80.

Diuretic. A drug that promotes the excretion of water through the urine.

Electrocardiogram (ECG or EKG). Record of the heart's electrical impulses.

Embolus. Blood clot that forms in one part of the body and is carried to another part of the body through the blood vessels.

Endothelium. Smooth layer of cells lining the heart (endocardium), blood vessels, and lymph vessels.

Enzyme. A complex chemical capable of initiating and speeding up specific biochemical processes in the body.

Epinephrine. A hormone released by the adrenal glands that speeds up heart rate and cardiac output. This in turn elevates blood pressure. Also called *adrenaline*.

Essential fatty acids (EFAs). Two classes of beneficial fats—omega-3 and omega-6 EFAs—that form cellular membranes, help the body absorb vitamins, and are the building blocks for many of the body's hormones. Fish oils and flaxseed and vegetable oils are rich sources of EFAs.

Free radical. An atom or molecule with an unpaired electron that is highly unstable and damaging to other molecules. Free radicals are neutralized by antioxidants.

Garlic. A medicinal and culinary herb (*Allium sativum*) used in the treatment of hypertension, hypercholesterolemia, and other disorders.

Heart attack. Damage or death to part of the heart muscle as a result of an insufficient blood supply. Also called *myocardial infarction.*

Heavy metal antagonist. An element, such as the trace mineral zinc, that can remove traces of lead, cadmium, and other heavy metals from the body.

High blood pressure. Blood pressure that is chronically elevated beyond the normal range. Also called *hypertension.*

High-density lipoprotein (HDL). Cholesterol carrier that transports cholesterol away from the tissues and to the liver so the cholesterol can be removed from the bloodstream. Sometimes called "good" cholesterol.

Hypertension. Blood pressure that is chronically elevated beyond the normal range. Also called *high blood pressure.*

Hypertensive nephrosclerosis. Stiffening and loss of elasticity of the arteries that supply blood to the kidneys, causing kidney malfunction.

Insulin-dependent diabetes mellitus. A type of diabetes in which the body cannot make its own supply of insulin. Also known as *type I diabetes.*

Insulin resistance. A condition in which insulin is unable to properly usher nutrients into the cells, leading to elevated blood levels of insulin and often to elevated levels of glucose. The underlying cause of syndrome X (see below).

Ischemic heart disease. Heart ailment caused by narrowed coronary arteries and characterized by a diminished blood supply to the heart. Also known as *coronary artery disease* and *coronary heart disease.*

Lipid. Fatty substance that is insoluble in blood.

Lipoprotein. Combination of a fatty substance surrounded by a protein.

Lipoprotein a (Lp[a]). A small particle that resembles LDL cholesterol; it sticks to small areas of damaged artery and initiates deadly blockages of the artery.

Low-density lipoprotein (LDL). Carrier of damaging cholesterol in the blood. Also known as "bad" cholesterol.

Mitral valve. Heart valve between the left ventricle and left atrium.

Monounsaturated fat. Type of fat found primarily in canola, olive, and walnut oil and avocados.

Muscular pump. The contraction and relaxation of the skeletal muscles that moves venous blood toward the heart.

Myocardial infarction. Damage or death to part of the heart muscle as a result of an insufficient blood supply; a heart attack.

Myocardium. Muscular wall of the heart that contracts to pump blood out of the heart and relaxes to refill the heart with returning blood.

Nephrons. Specialized ducts or funnels in the kidneys that act as monitoring stations, directing substances back into the blood or out of the body.

Non-insulin-dependent diabetes mellitus. A type of diabetes directly associated with syndrome X (see below) and specifically with extreme insulin resistance (see above). Also known as *type II diabetes* or *maturity-onset diabetes.*

Norepinephrine. A hormone released by the adrenal glands that constricts the blood vessels and raises the blood pressure. Also a neurotransmitter manufactured in the brain.

Obesity. Condition of significant overweight. Obesity strains the heart and increases chances of developing hypertension and diabetes.

Phytochemicals. A class of nutrients occurring naturally in plants; many have medicinal, health-enhancing properties.

Plaque. Fatty deposit lining the interior artery wall. Also called *atheroma.*

Plasma lipids. Fatty particles in the blood.

Platelets. One of the three types of blood-clotting elements found in the blood.

Polyunsaturated fats. Oils that are liquid at room temperature, including most vegetable oils, such as corn, sunflower, soybean, or safflower oil.

Primary hypertension. High blood pressure resulting mainly from poor dietary and lifestyle habits. Also called *essential hypertension.*

Renin. An enzyme released by the kidneys under conditions of stress, exercise, or certain changes in diet. Together with angiotensinogen, renin forms angiotensin I and initiates the RAAS (see below).

Renin-angiotensin-aldosterone system (RAAS). A potent hormone group whose primary function is to constrict blood vessels and increase arterial pressure.

Respiratory pump. The pressure changes that occur within your body when you breathe, which suck blood upward and help move blood along in the venous system.

Risk factors. Conditions that increase one's chances of developing a disease.

Saturated fats. Fats that are solid at room temperature, most commonly found in animal protein foods and tropical oils.

Secondary hypertension. High blood pressure resulting from an underlying physiological condition.

Sodium. A mineral found in nearly all plant and animal tissue. Table salt (sodium chloride) is almost half sodium.

Sodium-potassium pump. The shifting of sodium and potassium across cell membranes, which creates electricity and is the driving force of muscles, organs, and many bodily functions.

Sphygmomanometer. An instrument for measuring blood pressure. Consists of an inflatable arm cuff attached to a column of mercury and a gauge.

Stethoscope. A medical device for hearing sounds within the body.

Stress. Physical or mental tension related to external, biochemical, or emotional factors.

Stress response. Physiological reaction to a perceived threat that readies the body for "fight or flight." Involves hormones released by the hypothalamus, pituitary gland, and adrenal glands. Also called the *general adaptation syndrome.*

Stress test. A simple, painless diagnostic procedure, usually conducted on a treadmill or stationary bike in a doctor's office. While you exercise, several monitors measure your vital signs, and your physician uses the data to determine your fitness level. Recommended before you start a new exercise regimen.

Stroke. Sudden insufficient supply of blood to an area of the brain, sometimes resulting in loss of speech, muscle function, vision, or sensation. Also called *apoplexy, cerebrovascular accident,* or *cerebral vascular accident.*

Sudden death. Unexpected and instantaneous death, or the onset of death shortly after the experience of symptoms. The most common cause of sudden death is heart attack.

Syndrome X. A symptom complex identified by the presence of obesity (especially in the abdominal area), insulin resistance, elevated triglycerides, low HDL cholesterol, high blood pressure, high incidence of diabetes, and increased risk of heart disease.

Systolic blood pressure. Blood pressure measured in the arteries when the heart contracts. This is the first, or top, number in a blood pressure reading such as 120/80.

Thrombosis. Formation or presence of a blood clot (thrombus) inside a blood vessel or heart cavity.

Ubiquinone. See **Coenzyme Q10**.

Ultrasound. High-frequency, inaudible sound waves used for medical diagnosis.

Vascular. Pertaining to blood vessels.

Vein. Blood vessel returning blood from the body back to the heart.

Ventricular tachycardia. Condition in which the ventricle area of the heart produces a very fast, abnormal heartbeat.

Venule. Smaller blood vessel that branches off a vein.

White-coat hypertension. Temporarily elevated blood pressure resulting from the anxiety of being in a clinical setting and interacting with a health care professional.

Xenobiotic agents. Agents that are foreign to life. Modern drugs are xenobiotic because they are not natural compounds.

References

ALCOHOL AND BLOOD PRESSURE

Beilin, L. J., Puddey, I. B., Burke, V. (1996). "Alcohol and hypertension: Kill or cure?" *Journal of Hypertension* 10 (Suppl. 2), S1–S5.

Klatsky, A. L. et al. (1977). "Alcohol consumption and blood pressure." *New England Journal of Medicine* 296, 1194–1200.

MacMahon, S. (1987). "Alcohol consumption and hypertension." *Hypertension* 9 (2), 111–21.

Palmer, A. J. et al. (1995). "Alcohol intake and cardiovascular mortality in hypertensive patients: Report from the Department of Health Hypertension Care Computing Project." *Journal of Hypertension* 13, 957–64.

Randin, D. (1995). "Suppression of alcohol-induced hypertension of dexamethasone." *New England Journal of Medicine* 332, 1733–37.

Victor, R. G. and Hansen, M. (1995). "Alcohol and blood pressure—one drink a day." *New England Journal of Medicine* 332, 1782–83.

DIET, OBESITY AND WEIGHT LOSS, AND HYPERTENSION

Armstrong, B. (1977). "Blood pressure in Seventh Day Adventist." *American Journal of Epidemiology* 105, 444.

Burr, M. L. et al. (1981). "Plasma cholesterol and blood pressure in vegetarians." *Journal of Human Nutrition* 35, 437.

Friedman, M. (1976). "Effect of unsaturated fats upon lipemia and conjunctival circulation." *Journal of the American Medical Association* 198, 882.

———. (1984). "Serum lipids and conjunctival circulation after fat ingestion." *Circulation* 29, 874.

Gower, J. D. (1988). "A role for dietary lipids and antioxidants in the activation of carcinogens." *Free Radical Biology and Medicine* 5, 95–111.

Higgins, M. et al. (1993). "Benefits and adverse effects of weight loss: Observations from the Framingham Study." *Annual Internal Medicine* 7 (Part 2), 758–63.

Hollenberg, N. K. (1991). "Management of hypertension and cardiovascular risk." *American Journal of Medicine* 90 (Suppl. 2A), 2S–6S.

Kaplan, N. M. (1991). "Cardiovascular risk reduction: The role of antihypertensive treatment." *American Journal of Medicine* 90 (Suppl. 2A) 19S–20S.

Kempner, W. (1948). "Treatment of hypertensive vascular disease with rice diet." *American Journal of Medicine* 4, 545–77.

Klimes, I. et al. (1995). "The importance of diet therapy in the prevention and treatment of manifestations of metabolic syndrome X." *Vnitrni LeKarstvi* 41 (2), 136–40.

Ma, J. et al. (1995). "Associations of serum and dietary magnesium with cardiovascular disease, hypertension, diabetes, insulin, and carotid arterial wall thickness: The ARIC study." *Journal of Clinical Epidemiology* 48, 927–40.

Mahan, K. L. et al. (1996). *Escott-Stump, S. Krause's Food, Nutrition, and Diet Therapy* 9th ed. Philadelphia: W. B. Saunders, 108, 118, 338–39.

Nissinen, A. et al. (1989). "Unbalanced diets as a cause of chronic disease." *American Journal of Clinical Nutrition* 49 (Suppl. 5), 993–98.

Ozono, R. et al. (1995). "Systemic magnesium deficiency disclosed by magnesium loading test in patients with essential hypertension." *Hypertension Research* 18, 39–42.

Pennington, J. et al. (1991). "Total diet study: Nutritional elements, 1982–1989." *Journal of the American Dietetic Association* 91, 179–83.

Prigogine, I. and Stenger, L. (1984). *Order out of Chaos: Man's New Dialogue with Nature*. New York: Bantam.

Sacks, F. M. (1974). "Blood pressure in vegetarians." *American Journal of Epidemiology* 100, 390.

Sacks, F. M. et al. (1995). "Rationale and design of the Dietary Approaches to Stop Hypertension trial (DASH): A multicenter controlled-feedling study of dietary patterns to lower blood pressure." *Annals of Epidemiology* 5, 108–18.

Schotte, D. E. et al. (1990). "The effects of weight reduction on blood pressure in 301 obese patients." *Archives of Internal Medicine* 159 (8), 1701–4.

Subar, A. F. et al. (1995). "Fruit and vegetable intake in the United States: The baseline survey of the five a day for better health program." *American Journal of Health Promotion* 9 (5), 352–60.

Weber, M. A. (1989). "Antihypertensive treatment: Considerations beyond blood pressure control." *Circulation* 80 (6) (Suppl. M), IV–1204V–127.

Whyte, H. M. (1958). "Body fat and blood pressure of natives in New Guinea: Reflections on essential hypertension." *Australian Annals of Medicine* 7, 36–46.

Wilhelmsen, L. (1989). "Risks of untreated hypertension." *Hypertension* 13 (5) (Suppl. 5), 133–35.

Zusman, R. M. (1986). "Editorial: Alternatives to traditional antihypertensive therapy." *Hypertension* 8 (10), 837–42.

NUTRITIONAL THERAPIES

Auer, W. et al. (1990). "Hypertension and hyperlipidaemia: Garlic helps in mild cases." *British Journal of Clinical Practice Symposium Supplement* 69, 3–6.

Augusti, K. T. et al. (1996). "Antiperoxide effects of S-allyl cysteine sulfoxide, and insulin secretagogue, in diabetic rats." *Experientia* 52 (2), 115–20.

Ayback, M. et al. (1995). "Effect on oral pyridoxine hydrochloride supplementation on arterial blood pressure in patients with essential hypertension." *Arzneim Forsch* 45, 1271–73.

Bao, D. Q. et al. (1998). "Effects of dietary fish and weight reduction on ambulatory blood pressure in overweight hypertensives." *Hypertension* 32 (4), 710.

Bendich, A. et al. (1988). "Safety of beta-carotene." *Nutritional Cancer* 11, 207–14.

———. (1990). "Safety of vitamin A." *American Journal of Clinical Nutrition* 49, 358–71.

Braverman, E. R. (1995). *How to Lower Your Blood Pressure and Reverse Heart Disease Naturally*. Princeton, NJ: Publications for Achieving Total Health.

Casino, P. R. (1993). "The role of nitric oxide in endothelium-dependent vasodilation of hypercholesterolemic patients." *Circulation* 88 (6), 2541–7.

Cooke, J. P. (1998). "Is atherosclerosis an arginine deficiency disease?" *Journal of Investigative Medicine* 46 (8), 377–80.

Chytil, F. (1992). "The lungs and vitamin A." *American Journal of Physiology* 262, L517–L527.

Colette, C. et al. (1988). "Platelet function in type I diabetes: Effects of supplementation with large doses of vitamin E." *American Journal of Nutrition* 47, 256–61.

Digiesi, V. et al. (1994). "Coenzyme Q10 in essential hypertension." *Molecular Aspects of Medicine* 15, 57–63.

Dyckner, T. et al. (1983). "Effect of magnesium on blood pressure." *British Medical Journal* 286, 1847–49.

Engstrom, J. E. et al. (1992). "Vitamin C intake and mortality among a sample of the United States population." *Epidemiol* 3, 194–202.

Estrada, C. A. et al. (1993). "Patient preferences for novel therapy: An N-of-1 trial of garlic in the treatment for hypertension." *Journal of General Internal Medicine* 8, 619–21.

Fried, R. and Merrell, W. C. (1999). *The Arginine Solution*. New York: Warner Books.

Godin, D. V. et al. (1988). "Nutritional deficiency, starvation, and tissue and antioxidant status." *Free Radical Biology & Medicine* 5, 165–76.

Grossman, E. et al. (1996). "Should a moratorium be placed on sublingual nifedipine capsules given for hypertensive emergencies and pseudoemergencies?" *Journal of the American Medical Association* 276, 1328–31.

Heffner, J. E. and Repine, J. E. (1989). "Pulmonary strategies of antioxidant defenses." *American Review of Respiratory Disease* 140, 531–54.

Jain, S. K. and Wise, R. (1995). "Relationship between elevated lipid peroxides, vitamin E deficiency and hypertension in preeclampsia." *Molecular Cell Biochemistry* 151, 33–38.

Keli, S. O. et al. (1996). "Dietary flavonoids, antioxidant vitamins, and incidence of stroke." *Archives of Internal Medicine* 154, 637–42.

Kennedy, S. and Rice, D. A. (1992). "Histopathologic and ultrastructural myocardial alterations in calves deficient in vitamin E and selenium and fed polyunsaturated fatty acids." *Veterinary Pathology* 29, 129–38.

Korpela, H. et al. (1989). "Effect of selenium supplementation after acute myocardial infarction." *Research Communications in Chemical Pathology and Pharmacology* 65, 249–52.

Kushi, L. H. et al. (1996). "Dietary antioxidant vitamins and death from coronary heart disease in postmenopausal women." *New England Journal of Medicine* 18, 1156–62.

Langsjoen, P. et al. (1994). "Treatment of essential hypertension with coenzyme Q10." *Molecular Aspects of Medicine* 15 (Suppl.), S265–72.

Lee, W. H. (1983). *Kelp, Dulse and Other Sea Supplements.* New Canaan, CT: Keats Publishing, 1–9.

Losonczy, K. G. et al. (1996). "Vitamin E and vitamin C supplement use and risk of all-cause and coronary heart disease mortality in older persons: The established populations for epidemiologic studies of the elderly." *American Journal of Clinical Nutrition* 64, 190–96.

Mark, S. D. et al. (1996). "Lowered risks of hypertension and cerebrovascular disease after vitamin/mineral supplementation: The Linxian Nutrition Intervention Trial." *American Journal of Epidemiology* 143 (7), 658–64.

Maurer, I. et al. (1990). "Coenzyme Q10 and respiratory chain enzyme activities in hypertrophied human left ventricles with aortic valve stenosis." *American Journal of Cardiology* 66, 504–5.

McCarron, D. A. et al. (1984). "Blood pressure and nutrient intake in the United States." *Science* 224, 1392–98.

McCully, K. S. (1997). *The Homocysteine Revolution.* New Canaan, CT: Keats Publishing.

McNeill, J. H. et al. (1996). "Enhanced in vivo sensitivity of vanadyl-treated diabetic rats to insulin." *Canadian Journal of Physiology and Pharmacology* 68 (4), 486–91, 1990.

Meydani, M. (1992). "Modulation of the platelet thromboxane A2 and aortic prostacyclin synthesis by dietary selenium and vitamin E." *Biology and Trace Element Research* 33, 79.

Miura, S. et al. (1995). "Effects of various natural antioxidants on the Cu(2+)-mediated oxidative modification of low density lipoprotein." *Biological and Pharmacology Bulletin* 18 (1), 1–4.

Murray, M. T. (1997). *Heart Disease and High Blood Pressure.* Rocklin, CA: Prima Publishing.

Oberley, L. W. (1988). "Free radicals and diabetes." *Free Radical Biology and Medicine* 5, 113–24.

Public Health Service, DHHS (1988). Surgeon General's Report on Nutrition and Health. Publ. No. 88-50211.

Rapola, J. M. et al. (1996). "Effect of vitamin E and beta-carotene on the incidence of angina pectoris: A randomized double-blind, controlled trial." *Journal of the American Medical Association* 275 (9), 693–98.

Rayner, T. E. and Howe, P. R. (1995). "Purified omega-3 fatty acids retard the development of proteinuria in salt-loaded hypertensive rats." *Journal of Hypertension* 13, 771–80.

Riemersma, R. et al. (1991). "Risk of angina pectoris and plasma concentrations of vitamins A, C, and E and carotene." *Lancet* 337 (8732), 1–5.

Rimm, E. B. et al. (1993). "Vitamin E consumption and the risk of coronary heart disease." *New England Journal of Medicine* 328 (20), 1450–56.

Russo, C. et al. (1998). "Anti-oxidant status and lipid peroxidation in patients with essential hypertension." *Journal of Hypertension* 16, 1267–71.

Soloman, S. J. et al. (1983). "Effect of low zinc intake on carbohydrate and fat metabolism in men." *Federal Proceedings* 42, 391.

Somer, E. (June 1996). Nutrition Alert 96 Conference.

van Poppel, G. (1993). "Effect of beta-carotene on immunological indexes in healthy male smokers." *American Journal of Clinical Nutrition* 57, 402–7.

Vanderpas, J. B. (1990). "Iodine and selenium deficiency associated with cretinism in Northern Zaire." *American Journal of Clinical Nutrition* 52, 1087–93.

Washko, P. (1991). "Ascorbic acid in human neutrophils." *American Journal of Clinical Nutrition* 54, 1221S–7S.

Watson, R. et al. (1991). "Effect of beta-carotene on lymphocyte subpopulations in elderly humans: Evidence for a dose-response relationship." *American Journal of Clinical Nutrition* 53, 90.

Wen, Y. et al. (1996). "Lipid peroxidation and antioxidant vitamins C and E in hypertensive patients." *Irish Journal of Medical Science* 165 (3), 210–12.

Witteman, J. C. W. et al. (1994). "Reduction of blood pressure with oral magnesium supplementation in women with mild to moderate hypertension." *American Journal of Clinical Nutrition* 60, 129–35.

OTHER THERAPIES

Anshevevich, I. V. et al. (1985). "Serum aldosterone level in patients with hypertension during treatment by acupuncture." *Terapeuricheskii Arkhiv* 57 (10), 42–45.

Chappell, T. (1995). *Questions from the Heart.* Charlottesville, VA: Hampton Roads Publishing Company, Inc.

Chiu, Y. J. et al. (1997). "Cardiovascular and endocrine effects of acupuncture in hypertensive patients." *Clinical and Experiential Hypertension* 19 (7), 1047–63.

Meltzer, L. E. (April 1963). "Report on therapy, the treatment of coronary artery disease with disodium EDTA, a reappraisal." *American Journal of Cardiology,* 501.

Olszewer, E. et al. (1988). "EDTA chelation therapy in chronic degenerative disease." *Medical Hypotheses* 27, 41–49.

COGNITIVE DYSFUNCTION

DeCarli, C. et al. (1999). "Predictors of brain morphology for the men of the NHLBI twin study." *Stroke* 30 (3), 529–36.

Glynn, R. J. et al. (1999). "Current and remote blood pressure and cognitive decline." *Journal of the American Medical Association* 281 (5), 438–45.

Snowdon, D. A. et al. (1997). "Brain infarction and the clinical expression of Alzheimer Disease." *Journal of the American Medical Association* 277 (10), 813–17.

CARDIOVASCULAR DISEASES

American Heart Association (March 11, 1997). High blood pressure prematurely "ages" blood vessels' linings, new study shows. www.americanheart.org

Cruickshank, J. M. (1988). "Coronary flow reserve and the J curve relation between diastolic blood pressure and myocardial infarction." *British Medical Journal* 297, 1227–30.

Felicetta, F. V. (1996). "Hypertension in the elderly." *Clinical Geriatrics* 4 (10), 87–93.

Holienberg, N. K. (1987). "Cardiovascular therapeutics in the 1980s: An ounce of prevention." *American Journal of Medicine* 82 (Suppl. 3A), 1–3.

Kannel, W. B. (1995). "Framingham study insights into hypertensive risk of cardiovascular disease." *Hypertension Research* 18, 181–96.

Kaplan, N. (1995). "The treatment of hypertension in women." *Archives of Internal Medicine* 155, 563–67.

Keli, S. et al. (1992). "Predictive value of repeated systolic blood pressure measurements for stroke risk: The Zutphen study." *Stroke* 23 (3), 347–51.

Launer, L. J. et al. (1995). "The association between midlife blood pressure levels and late-life cognitive function." *Journal of the American Medical Association* 274 (23), 1846–51.

Leren, P. et al. (1986). "Coronary heart disease and treatment of hypertension: Some Oslo Study data." *American Journal of Medicine* 80 (Suppl. 2A), 3–6.

MacMahon, S. et al. (1990). "Blood pressure, stroke, and coronary heart disease. Part 1: Prolonged differences in blood pressure; prospective observational studies corrected for the regression dilution bias." *Lancet* 335, 765–74.

Monte, T. (1993). *World Medicine, the East West Guide to Healing Your Body.* New York: Jeremy P. Tarcher/Perigee Books.

National Health and Nutrition Examination Survey II (NHANES II), 1976–80, and the American Heart Association.

National Health and Nutrition Examination Survey III, Phase I, (NHANES III), 1988–91, and the American Heart Association.

National High Blood Pressure Education Program, National Heart, Lung, and Blood Institute and the National Institutes of Health (1979). "What every woman should know about high blood pressure," 287–447.

Pang, P. K. et al. (1996). "Parathyroid hypertensive factor and intracellular calcium regulation." *Journal of Hypertension* 14, 1053–60.

Russell, M. A. (1969–1990). "Age-specific patterns of mortality from cardiovascular disease and other major causes." *Australian Journal of Public Health* 18, 160–64.

Skoog, I. (1996). "Fifteen-year longitudinal study of blood pressure and dementia." *Lancet* 347, 1131–45.

Taddei, S. et al. (1997). "Hypertension causes premature aging of endothelial function in humans." *Hypertension* 29 (3), 736–43.

Vasan, B. S. et al. (1996). "The role of hypertension in the pathogenesis of heart failure." *Archives of Internal Medicine* 156, 1789–96.

Weinberger, M. H. (1988). "Cardiovascular risk factors and antihypertensive therapy." *American Journal of Medicine* 84 (Suppl. 4A), 24–29.

Wilhelmsen, L. (1989). "Risks of untreated hypertension." *Hypertension* (Suppl. I), 13 (5), I-33–34.

The Working Group on Hypertension in the Elderly (1986). Statement on hypertension in the elderly. *Journal of the American Medical Association* 256, 70–74.

DRUGS AND MEDICAL ECONOMICS

Alderman, M. H., Ooi, W. L., Madhavan, S., Cohen, H. (1989). "Treatment-induced blood pressure reduction and the risk of myocardial infarction." *Journal of the American Medical Association* 262, 920–24.

Ambard, L. and Beaujard, (1904). "Causes de l'hypertension arterielle." *Archives of General Medicine* (Paris) 81, 520–33.

Ames, R. P. (1983). "Negative effects of diuretic drugs on metabolic risk factors for coronary heart disease: Possible alternative drug therapies." *American Journal of Cardiology* 51, 632–38.

Breckenridge, A. (1985). "Editorial accompanying British MRC report. Treating mild hypertension." *British Journal of Medicine* 291, 89–97.

Carb, J. D. et al. (1985). "Long-term surveillance for adverse effects of antihypertensive drugs." *Journal of the American Medical Association* 253, 3263–68.

Carpi, J. (1995). "Calcium channel blocker debate refuses to die." *Internal Medicine News* 28 (12), 1.

Chait, A. (1989). "Effects of antihypertensive agents on serum lipids and lipoproteins." *American Journal of Medicine* 86 (Suppl. 1 B), 5–7.

Cohen, A. M., Senate Hearings, April 30, 1973.

Collins, R. et al. (1990). "Blood pressure, stroke, and coronary heart disease. Part 2. Short-term reductions in blood pressure: Overview of randomized drug trials in their epidemiological context." *Lancet* 335, 827–38.

Conway, Jennifer, ed. (1986). "Studies reveal prescribing trend in hypertension adds to healthcare inflation." *LDI News*, Philadelphia, PA.

Edmonds, C. J. and Janasi, B. (1972). "Total-body potassium in hypertensive patients during prolonged diuretic therapy." *Lancet* 2, 8–12.

Flamenbaum, W. (1983). "Metabolic consequences of antihypertensive therapy." *Annals of Internal Medicine* 98, 875–80.

Furberg, C. D. et al. (1995). "Dose-related increase in mortality in patients with coronary heart disease." *Circulation* 91, 2855–56.

Ginzberg, E. (November 12, 1992). "The health swamp." *New York Times,* A25.

Gorelick, P. B. (1995). "Stroke prevention." *Archive of Neurology* 52 (4), 347–55.

Helgeland, A. (1980). "Treatment of mild hypertension: A five year controlled drug trial—The Oslo Study." *American Journal of Medicine* 69, 725–32.

Hiatt, W., Stoll, S., Nies, A. (1985). "Effect of beta-adrenergic blockers on the peripheral circulation in patients with peripheral vascular disease." *Circulation* 72, 1226–31.

Hypertension Detection and Follow-up Program Cooperative Group (1982). "The effect of treatment on mortality in 'mild' hypertension." *New England Journal of Medicine* 307 (16), 976–80.

Jachuck, S. J. et al. (1982). "The effects of hypotensive drugs on the quality of life." *Journal of the College of General Practitioners* 32, 103.

Johnson, J. A. and Bootman, J. L. (1995). "Drug-related morbidity and mortality: A cost-of-illness model." *Archives of Internal Medicine* 155, 1949–56.

Julius, S. et al. (1990). "The association of borderline hypertension with target organ changes and higher coronary risk: Tecumseh blood pressure study." *Journal of the American Medical Association* 264, 354–58.

Kessler, D. A. et al. (1990). "The federal regulation of prescription drug advertising and promotion." *Journal of the American Medical Association* 264 (18), 2409–15.

Lassen, C. et al. (1991). "Computerized surveillance of adverse drug events in hospital patients." *Journal of the American Medical Association* 226 (20), 2847–51.

Lazarou, J. et al. (1998). "Incidence of adverse drug reactions in hospitalized patients." *Journal of the American Medical Association* 279 (15), 1200–1205.

Leren, P. et al. (1980). "Effect of propranolol and prazosin on blood lipids. The Oslo study." *Lancet* 2, 4–6.

Levin, E. et al. (1985). "Case report: Severe hypertension induced by naloxone." *American Journal of Medical Science* 290, 70–72.

Manolio, T. A. et al. (1995). "Trends in pharmacologic management of hypertension in the United States." *Archives of Internal Medicine* 155, 829–34.

McCarron, D. A. et al. (1984). "Therapeutic and economic controversies in antihypertensive therapy." *Journal of Cardiovascular Pharmacology* 6, S837–40.

Medical Research Council Working Party (1985). "MRC trial of treatment of mild hypertension: Principal results." *British Journal of Medicine* 291, 97–104.

Morgan, T. O. et al. (1980). "Failure of therapy to improve prognosis in elderly males with hypertension." *Medical Journal of Australia* 2, 27–31.

Multiple Risk Factor Intervention Trial Research Group (1982). "Multiple risk factor intervention trial. Risk factor changes and mortality results." *Journal of the American Medical Association* 248 (12), 1465–77.

Neergaard, L. (July 11, 1998). "Critics question FDA after drug bans." *Orange County Register.*

Nordrehaug, J. E. and von der Lippe, G. (1983). "Hypokalaemia and ventricular fibrillation in acute myocardial infarction." *British Heart Journal* 50, 525–29.

Oliver, M. P. (1982). "Risks of correcting the risks of coronary disease and stroke with drugs." *New England Journal of Medicine* 306 (5), 297–98.

Pahor, M. et al. (1996). "Calcium-channel blockade and incidence of cancer affected populations." *Lancet* 348 (9026), 487.

Physicians' Desk Reference, 48th ed. (1994). Oradell, NJ: Medical Economics Data.

"Propose demoting diuretics from 'No. 1' in HBP step care." (1983). Medical Tribune 5 (25), 6.

Psaty, B. M. et al. (1994). "The risk of incident myocardial infarction associated with antihypertensive drug therapies [abstract]." *Circulation* 91 (3), 925.

———. (1995). "The risk of myocardial infarction associated with antihypertensive drug therapies." *Journal of the American Medical Association* 274, 620–25.

Schoenberger, J. A. (1988). "New approaches to a first-line treatment of hypertension." *American Journal of Medicine* 84 (Suppl. 3B), 26–31.

Sesoko, S. and Kaneko, Y. (1985). "Cough associated with the use of captopril." *Archives of Internal Medicine* 145, 1524.

Sheps, S. G. (1999). *Mayo Clinic on High Blood Pressure.* Rochester, MN: Mayo Clinic.

Smith, W. M., Edlavitch, S. C., Krushalt, W. (1979). "U.S. Public Health Service Hospitals intervention trial in mild hypertension." In G. Onesti and C. R. Klimt (Eds.), *Hypertension-determinants, Complications and Intervention.* New York: Grune and Stratton.

Smith, W. M. (1977). "Treatment of mild hypertension. Results of a ten-year intervention trial." *Circulation Review* 40 (Suppl. 1), I98–I105.

Stallones, R. A., Dyken, M. L., Fang, H. C. (1972). "Epidemiology for stroke facilities planning." *Stroke* 3, 360.

Stason, W. B. (1989). "Cost and quality tradeoffs in the treatment of hypertension." *Hypertension* 13 (Suppl. 1), 145–48.

U.S. Department of Health and Human Services, Public Health Service, National Center for Health Statistics. Blood pressure levels in persons 18–74 years of age in 1976–1980 in the United States.

Veterans Administration Cooperative Study Group on Antihypertensive Agents (1967). "Effects of treatment on morbidity in hypertension I. Results in patients with diastolic blood pressures averaging 115 through 129 mm Hg." *Journal of the American Medical Association* 202, 1028–34.

———. (1970). "Effects of treatment on morbidity in hypertension II. Results in patients with diastolic blood pressures averaging 90 through 114 mm Hg." *Journal of the American Medical Association* 213, 114-3–52.

———. (1987). "Comparison of propranalol and hydrochlorothiazide for the initial treatment of hypertension. Results of long-term therapy." *Journal of the American Medical Association* 248, 2 (4–1).

Wilcox, R. B., Mitchell, J. R. A., Hampton, J. R. (1986). "Treatment of high blood pressure: Should clinical practice be based on results of clinical trials?" *British Journal of Medicine* 293, 433–37.

Wilkinson, P. R. et al. (1975). "Total body and serum potassium during prolonged thiazide therapy for essential hypertension." *Lancet* 1, 759–62.

Wordsworth, B. and Mowat, A. (1985). "Raid development of gout tophi after diuretic therapy." *Journal of Rheumatism* 12, 376–77.

Zawada, E. T. (1989). "Metabolic considerations in the approach to diabetic hypertensive patients." *American Journal of Medicine* 87 (Suppl. 6A), 34S–38S.

EXERCISE/LIFESTYLE

American College of Sports Medicine (1993). "Position stand physical activity, physical fitness, and hypertension." *Medical Science Sports Exercise* 10, i–x.

Araujo-Vilar, D. et al. (1997). "Influence of moderate physical exercise on insulin-medicated and non-insulin-medicated glucose uptake in healthy subjects." *Metabolism Clinical and Experimental* (46) 2, 203–9.

Batmanghelidj, F. (1995). *Your Body's Many Cries for Water.* Falls Church, VA: Global Health Solutions, Inc.

Bertrand, E., Frances, Y., Lafay, V. (1995). "Physical training and blood pressure." *Bulletin de l'Academie Nationale Medicine* 179 (7), 1471–80.

Cade, R. et al. (1984). "Effect of aerobic exercise training on patients with systemic arterial hypertension." *American Journal of Medicine* 77, 785–90.

Gordon, G. (1997). "Interview with chelation pioneer." *Life Enhancement* 32, 7–15.

Hagberg, J. M. and Seals, D. R. (1986). "Exercise training and hypertension." *Acta Medica Scandinavica Supplementum* 711, 131–36.

Hagberg, J. M. et al. (1989). "Effect of exercise training in 60- to 69-year-old persons with essential hypertension." *American Journal of Cardiology* 64 (5), 348–53.

Halbert, J. A. et al. (1997). "The effectiveness of exercise training in lowering blood pressure: A meta-analysis of randomised controlled trials of 4 weeks or longer." *Journal of Hypertension* 11 (10), 641–49.

Henriksson, J. (1995). "Influence of exercise on insulin sensitivity." *Journal of Cardiovascular Risk* 4, 303–9.

Hollenberg, N. K. (1991). "Management of hypertension and cardiovascular risk." *American Journal of Medicine* 90 (Suppl. 2A), 2S–6S.

Kahle, E. B. et al. (1996). "Associations between mild, routine exercise and improved insulin dynamics and glucose control in obese adolescents." *International Journal of Sports Medicine* 1, 1–6.

Kaplan, N. M. (1991). "Cardiovascular risk reduction: The role of antihypertensive treatment." *American Journal of Medicine* 90 (Suppl. 2A), 19S–20S.

Kelley, G. A. (1989). "Aerobic exercise and resting blood pressure among women: A meta-analysis." *Preventive Medicine* 28 (3), 264–75.

———. (1995). "Effects of aerobic exercise in normotensive adults: A brief meta-analytic review of controlled clinical trials." *Southern Medical Journal* 88 (2), 42–46.

Kelley, G. A. et al. (1994). "Antihypertensive effects of aerobic exercise: A brief meta-analytic review of randomized controlled trials." *American Journal of Hypertension* 7 (2), 115–19.

Lauer, M. S. et al. (1995). "Angiographic and prognostic implications of an exaggerated exercise systolic blood pressure response and rest systolic blood pressure in adults undergoing evaluation for suspected coronary artery disease." *Journal of the American College of Cardiology* 26 (7), 1630–36.

Ornish, D. et al. (1990). "Can lifestyle changes reverse coronary heart disease? The Lifestyle Heart Trial." *Lancet* 336, 129–33.

Schwartz, R. S. (1995). "The effects of endurance and resistance training on blood pressure." *International Journal of Obesity and Related Metabolic Disorder* 10 (Suppl. 4), S52–57.

Stamlers, R. et al. (1989). "Primary prevention of hypertension by nutritional-hygienic means." *Journal of the American Medical Association* 262 (113), 1801–7.

SALT, HYPERTENSION, AND MINERAL BALANCE

Albert, D. G. et al. (1983). "Serum magnesium and plasma sodium levels in hypertension." *New England Journal of Medicine* 309, 888–91.

Altura, B. M. et al. (1983). "Magnesium deficiency-induced spasms of umbilical vessels: Relation to preeclampsia, hypertension, growth retardation." *Science* 221, 376–78.

———. (1984). "Magnesium deficiency and hypertension: Correlation between magnesium-deficient diets and microcirculatory changes in situ." *Science* 223, 1315–17.

Brancati, F. L. et al. (1996). "Effect of potassium supplementation on blood pressure in African Americans on a low-potassium diet." *Archives of Internal Medicine* 156, 61–67.

Bulpitt, C. J., Shipley, M. J., Semmence, A. (1981). "Blood pressure and plasma sodium and potassium." *Clinical Sciences* 61, 85S–87S.

Conn, J. W. (1949). "The mechanism of acclimatization to heat." *Advances in Internal Medicine* 3, 373–93.

Dahl, L. K. (1972). "Salt and hypertension." *American Journal of Clinical Nutrition* 25, 231–44.

Dyckner, T. and Wester, P. O. (1983). "Effects of magnesium on blood pressure." *British Journal of Medicine* 286, 1847–49.

———. (1987). "Potassium/magnesium depletion in patients with cardiovascular disease." *American Journal of Medicine* 82 (Suppl. 3A), 1–17.

Gimeno, O. A. et al. (1990). "Relationship of several physico-chemical components in drinking water, hypertension and cardiovascular disease mortality." *Revista de Sanidad e Higiene Publica* 64, 377–85.

Grim, C. E. et al. (1980). "Racial differences in blood pressure in Evans County, Georgia: Relationship to sodium and potassium intake and plasma renin activity." *Journal of Chronic Diseases* 33, 87–94.

Haddy, F. J. (1960). "Local effects of sodium, calcium, and magnesium upon small and large blood vessels of the dog forelimb." *Circulation Research* 8, 57–70.

Heiner, C. G. (1996). "Effects of dietary calcium supplementation on blood pressure." *Journal of the American Medical Association* 275, 1016–22.

Hollenberg, N. K. (1991). "Management of hypertension and cardiovascular risk." *American Journal of Medicine* 90 (Suppl. 2A), 2S–6S.

Houtman, J. P. (1996). "Trace elements and cardiovascular diseases." *Journal of Cardiovascular Risk* 1, 18–25.

Ito, Y. and Fujitar, T. (1996). "Trace elements and blood pressure regulation." *Nippon Rinsho* 54, 106–10.

Johnson, N. E. and Fujitar, T. (1985). "Effects on blood pressure of calcium supplementation of women." *American Journal of Clinical Nutrition* 42, 12–17.

Kaats, G. R. (1998). "Double-masked, placebo-controlled study of the effect of chromium picolinate supplementative on body composition: A replication and extension of a previous study." *Current Therapeutic Research* 59 (6), 379–88.

Krotkiewski, M. et al. (1995). "Mild hypertension treated with a sodium-potassium ion-exchanging seaweed preparation." *Cardiovascular Reviews and Reports* 11, 35–48.

Lim, P. and Jacob, E. (1972). "Magnesium deficiency in patients on long-term diuretic therapy for heart failure." *British Medical Journal* 9, 620–22.

Longnecker, M. P. (1991). "Selenium in diet, blood, and toenails in relation to human health in seleniferous area." *American Journal of Clinical Nutrition* 53, 1288–94.

Luft, F. C. and Weinberger, M. H. (1982). "Sodium intake and essential hypertension." *Hypertension* 4 (5), 14–19.

Ma, J. et al. (1995). "Associations of serum and dietary magnesium and cardiovascular disease, hypertension, diabetes, insulin, and carotid arterial wall thickness: The Atherosclerosis Risk in Communities Study." *Journal of Clinical Epidemiology* 48, 927–40.

MacGregor, G. A. et al. (1982). "Moderate potassium supplementation in essential hypertension." *Lancet* 8297, 567–70.

McCarron, D. A. (1982). "Low serum concentrations of ionized calcium in patients with hypertension." *New England Journal of Medicine* 307, 226–31.

————. (1997). "Role of adequate dietary calcium in the prevention of and management of salt-sensitive hypertension." *American Journal of Clinical Nutrition* (Suppl. 2), 712S–16S.

Moore, R. D. (1993). *The High Blood Pressure Solution.* Rochester, VT: Healing Arts Press.

Moore, R. D. and Webb, G. D. (1986). *The K Factor: Reversing and Preventing High Blood Pressure without Drugs.* New York: Macmillan.

Resnick, L. M. et al. (1983). "Divalent cations in essential hypertension." *New England Journal of Medicine* 309, 888–91.

Ross, S. (1995). "Calcium channel blockers." *Clinical Pharmacy Review* (PCS Health Systems), 1.

Sirving, O. et al. (1996). "Dietary flavonoids, antioxidant vitamins, and incidence of stroke." *Archives of Internal Medicine* 154, 637–42.

Srivastava, V. et al. (1993). "The significance of serum magnesium in diabetes mellitus." *Indian Journal of Medical Science* 46 (5).

Takagi, Y. et al. (1991). "Calcium treatment of essential hypertension in elderly patients evaluated by 24 H monitoring." *American Journal of Hypertension* 4, 836–39.

Tarek, F. T. et al. (1996). "Salt—more adverse effects." *Lancet* 348, 250–51.

Touyz, R. M. et al. (1995). "Relations between magnesium, calcium, and plasma renin activity in black and white hypertensive patients." *Minor Electrolyte Metabolism* 21, 417–22.

Usehima, H. et al. (1981). "Hypertension, salt, and potassium." *Lancet* 1, 504.

Weber, M. A. (1989). "Antihypertensive treatment: Considerations beyond blood pressure control." *Circulation* 80 (6) (Suppl. M), IV-1204V-127.

Young, D. R. et al. (1999). "The effects of aerobic exercise and T'ai Chi on blood pressure in older people: Results of a randomized trial." *Journal of the American Geriatric Society* 47 (3), 277–84.

Zusman, R. M. (1986). "Editorial: Alternative antihypertensive therapy." *Hypertension* 8, 837–42.

POTASSIUM

Intersalt Cooperative Research Group (1988). "Intersalt: An international study of electrolyte excretion and blood pressure. Results for 24-hour urinary sodium and potassium excretion." *British Journal of Medicine* 297, 319–28.

Morgan, T. et al. (1987). "Comparative studies of reduced sodium and high potassium diet in hypertension." *Nephron* 47 (Suppl. 1), 21–26.

Siani, A. et al. (1991). "Increasing the dietary potassium intake reduces the need for antihypertension medication." *Annals of Internal Medicine* 115, 753–59.

HYPERTENSION DETECTION AND RISK FACTORS

Batuman, V. et al. (1983). "Contribution of lead to hypertension with renal impairment." *New England Journal of Medicine* 309, 17–20.

Bland, J. S. (1999). *Improving Intercellular Communication in Managing Chronic Illness.* Gig Harbor, WA: HealthComm International, Inc.

Felknor, R. (1994). "New hypertension guidelines stress systolic pressure." *Cardiology World News,* 22–23.

Grossman, E. and Messerli, F. H. (1995). "High blood pressure: A side effect of drugs, poisons, and food." *Archives of Internal Medicine* 155, 450–60.

Gurwitz, J. H. (1994). "Initiation of antihypertensive treatment during nonsteroidal anti-inflammatory drug therapy." *Journal of the American Medical Association* 272, 781–86.

Hansson, L. et al. (1998). "Effects of intensive blood-pressure lowering and low-dose aspirin in patients with hypertension: Principal results of the Hypertension Optimal Treatment (HOT) randomized trial." *Lancet* 351, 1755–62.

Hu, H. (1991). "A 50 year follow-up of childhood plumbism: Hypertension, renal function, and hemoglobin levels among survivors." *American Journal of Diseases of Children* 145, 681–87.

Hu, H. et al. (1996). "The relationship of bone and blood lead to hypertension: The Normative Aging Study." *Journal of the American Medical Association* 275, 1171–76.

Hypertension Detection and Follow-up Program Cooperative Group (1979). "Five-year findings of the hypertension detection and follow-up program. II. Mortality by race, sex and age." *Journal of the American Medical Association* 242, 2562–77.

Joaquim de Oliveira, J. and Silva, S. R. (1996). "Arterial hypertension due to mercury intoxication with clinico-laboratorial syndrome simulating pheochromocytomal." *Arquious Brasileiros de Cardiologia* 66, 29–31.

Koop, C. E. (June 10, 1998). "The link between obesity and diseases [letter]." *Wall Street Journal.*

Krauss, R. M. (1991). "The tangled web of coronary risk factors." *American Journal of Medicine* 90 (Suppl. 2A), 36S–41S.

Le Pailleur, C. et al. (1998). "The effects of talking, reading, and silence on the 'white coat' phenomenon in hypertensive patients." *American Journal of Hypertension* 11 (2), 203–7.

Lu, K. P., Zhao, S. H., Wang, D. S. (1990). "The stimulatory effect of heavy metal cations on proliferation of aortic smooth muscle cells." *Science in China, Series B.* 33 (3), 303–10.

Management Committee (1981). "The Australian therapeutic trial in mild hypertension." *Lancet* 1, 1261–67.

Moser, M. et al. (1998). "Critique of treatment recommendations of the 6th Joint National Committee on Prevention, Detection, Evaluation and Treatment of Hypertension in special populations." *CVR&R,* 29–37.

Multiple Risk Factor Intervention Trial Research Group (1982). "Multiple Risk Factor Intervention Trial: Risk factor changes and mortality results." *Journal of the American Medical Association* 248, 1465–77.

Page, L. B., Damon, A., Moellering, R. C. (1974). "Jr. Antecedents of cardiovascular disease in six Solomon Island societies." *Circulation* 49, 1132–46.

Papademetriou, V. et al. (1998). "Management of hypertension with or without comorbidities." *Cardiology Special Edition* 4 (2), 9–13.

Pental, P. (1984). "Toxicity of over-the-counter stimulants." *Journal of the American Medical Association* 252, 1898–1903.

Reuters Health Information (February 19, 1998). Four personality profiles respond to diagnosis of hypertension differently. www.reutershealth.com

———. (February 4, 1999). New blood pressure guidelines: lower is better. www.reutershealth.com

———. (March 5, 1999). Morning caffeine raises blood pressure, adrenaline levels into evening. www.reutershealth.com

Saken, R. et al. (1979). "Drug-induced hypertension in infancy." *Journal of Pediatric Medicine* 95, 1077–79.

Schwartz, J. (1991). "Lead, blood pressure, and cardiovascular disease in men and women." *Environmental Health Perspective* 91, 71–75.

Sinclair, A. M. et al. (1987). "Secondary hypertension in blood pressure clinic." *Archives of Internal Medicine* 147, 1289–93.

Sternberg, E. B. et al. (1984). "Drugs that induce hypertension: A discussion of mechanisms." *Dateline Hypertension* 2 (4), 1–7.

"Tackling High Blood Pressure" (1989). *Nutrition Action,* 5, 5–7.

Tyroler, H. A. (1987). "Twenty-year mortality in black residents of Evans County, Georgia." *Journal of Clinical Hypertension* (Suppl. 3), 9–15.

Tzagournis, M. (1989). "Interaction of diabetes with hypertension—patients at high risk: An overview." *American Journal of Medicine* 86 (Suppl. 1B), 50–54.

Voors, A. W. et al. (1975). "Some determinants of blood pressure in children age 4–14 years in a total biracial community—the Bogalusa Heart Study." Presented before the Epidemiology Session at the American Heart Association 27th Annual Meeting. Anaheim, CA.

Weinberger, M. H. et al. (June 1996). "Sodium sensitivity and resistance of blood pressure in humans." Paper presented at the Institute of Food Technologists 46th Annual Meeting. Dallas, TX.

Working Group Report on Primary Prevention of Hypertension (1993). "National High Blood Pressure Education Program: National Heart, Lung, and Blood Institute." *Archives of Internal Medicine* 153, 186–208.

SMOKING AND BLOOD PRESSURE

Baer, L. and Rudichevich, I. (1985). "Cigarette smoking in hypertensive patients: Blood pressure and endocrine responses." *American Journal of Medicine* 78, 564–68.

Breckenridge, A. (1985). "Treating mild hypertension." *British Medical Journal (Clinical Research Edition)* 291 (6488), 89–90.

Medical Research Council Working Party (1985). "MRC trial of treatment of mild hypertension: Principal results." *British Medical Journal* 291, 97–104.

Working Group Report on Primary Prevention of Hypertension (1993). "National Blood Pressure Education Program: National Heart, Lung, and Blood Institute." *Archives of Internal Medicine* 153, 186–208.

STATISTICS AND GENERAL INFORMATION

American Heart Association (1996). Heart attack and stroke facts (1996 suppl.), Dallas, TX.

———. (1999). Cardiovascular Diseases. www.amhrt.org/statistics/03cardio.html

Cooper, R. S. et al. (1999). "The puzzle of hypertension in African-Americans." *Scientific American,* 56–63.

Fifth Report of the Joint National Committee on Detection, Evaluation, and Treatment of High Blood Pressure (1993). *Archives of Internal Medicine* 153, 154–83.

Grossman, E. and Messerli, F. (1995). "High blood pressure: A side effect of drugs, poisons and food." *Archives of Internal Medicine* 155, 450–60.

Hypertension Detection and Follow-up Program Cooperative Group (1979). "Five-year findings of the hypertension detection and follow-up program. I. Reduction in mortality of persons with high blood pressure, including mild hypertension. II. Mortality by race, sex and age." *Journal of the American Medical Association* 242, 2562–77.

Joint National Committee of Detection, Evaluation, and Treatment of High Blood Pressure (1988). *Archives of Internal Medicine* 148, 1023–103.

Kaplan, N. M. (1991). "Cardiovascular risk reduction: The role of antihypertensive treatment." *American Journal of Medicine* 90 (Suppl. 2A).

Kempner, W. (1948). "Treatment of hypertensive vascular disease with rice diet." *American Journal of Medicine* 4, 545–77.

Krauss, R. M. (1991). "The tangled web of coronary risk factors." *American Journal of Medicine* 90 (Suppl. 2A), 36S–41S.

Marieb, E. N. (1998). *Human Anatomy & Physiology.* Menlo Park, CA: Benjamin/Cummings Science Publishing.

Medical Research Council Working Party (1985). "MRC trial of treatment of mild hypertension: Principal results." *British Journal of Medicine* 291, 97–104.

Messerli, F. et al. (1988). "Effects of calcium channel blockers on systemic hemodynamics in hypertension." *American Journal of Medicine* 84 (Suppl. 3B), 8–12.

Moore, R. D. and Webb, G. D. (1986). *The K Factor. Reversing and Preventing High Blood Pressure without Drugs.* New York: Macmillan.

Murray, M. T. (1995). *The Healing Power of Herbs.* Rocklin, CA: Prima Publishing.

Newman, T. B. et al. (1996). "Carcinogenicity of lipid-lowering drugs." *Journal of the American Medical Association* 275 (1), 55–60.

Nissinen, A. and Stanley, K. (1989). "Unbalanced diets as a cause of chronic disease." *American Journal of Clinical Nutrition* 49, 993–98.

Olzewer, E. et al. (1988). "EDTA chelation therapy in chronic degenerative disease." *Medical Hypotheses* 27, 41–49.

Scandinavian Simvastatin Survival Study Group (November 1994). "Randomized trial of cholesterol lowering in 4444 patients with coronary heart disease." *The Scandinavian Survival Study (4S)* 344, 1383–89.

Selhub, J. (1995). "Association between plasma homocysteine concentrations and extracranial carotid-artery stenosis." *New England Journal of Medicine* 332 (5), 286–91.

Society of Actuaries and Association of Life Insurance Medical Directors of America. Blood Pressure Study 1979 and 1980.

Trials of Hypertension Prevention Collaborative Research Group (1992). "The effects of nonpharmacologic interventions on blood pressure of persons with high normal levels: Results of the Trials of Hypertension Prevention, Phase 1." *Journal of the American Medical Association* 267, 1213–20.

U.S. Public Health Service (1980). "The 1980 report of the Joint National Committee on Detection, Evaluation, and Treatment of High Blood Pressure." NIH Publication No. 81-1098, Washington, DC: U.S. Department of Health and Human Services.

———. (1984). "Third Report of the Joint National Committee of Detection, Evaluation, and Treatment of High Blood Pressure." *Archives of Internal Medicine* 144, 1045–57.

Verschurten, W. M. et al. (1995). "Serum total cholesterol and long-term coronary heart disease mortality in different cultures." *Journal of the American Medical Association* 274 (2), 131–36.

Waaler, H. T. and Holmen, J. (1991). "Systolic and diastolic blood-pressure values indicating equivalent risk." *New England Journal of Medicine* 325, 434–35.

Working Group Report on Primary Prevention of Hypertension (1993). "National High Blood Pressure Education Program: National Heart, Lung, and Blood Institute." *Archives of Internal Medicine* 153, 186–208.

STRESS REDUCTION

Anderson, D. E. et al. (1995). "Inhibited breathing decreases renal sodium excretion." *Psychological Medicine* 57, 373–80.

Benson, H. (1975). *The Relaxation Response.* New York: Avon Books.

Blaustien, M. P. (1977). "Sodium ions, calcium ions, blood pressure regulation, and hypertension. A reassessment and a hypothesis." *American Journal of Physiology* 232, C165–73.

Brewer, S. (1997). *High Blood Pressure.* London: Thorsons.

DiBona, G. F. (1991). "Stress and sodium intake in neural control of renal function in hypertension." *Hypertension* 17 (Suppl. 3), 2–5.

Hirsch, A. R. (1997). *Dr. Hirsch's Guide to Scentsational Weight Loss.* Rockport, MA: Element Books, Inc.

Markovitz, J. et al. (1993). "Psychological predictors of hypertension in the Framingham Study." *Journal of the American Medical Association* 370 (20), 2439–42.

Pickering, T. (1993). "Tension and hypertension." *Journal of the American Medical Association* 370, 2494.

Tisserand, R. (1995). "Aromatherapy as mind-body medicine." *International Journal of Aromatherapy* 6 (3), 14–19.

SYNDROME X AND INSULIN RESISTANCE

American Diabetes Association, Diabetes facts and figures. www.diabetes.org/ada

Bellenir, K. and Dresser, P. D., eds. (1994). *Diabetes Sourcebook Health Reference Series*, Vol. 3. Detroit, MI: Omnigraphics.

Block, W. (1997). "Carbohydrate-caused diabetes." *Life Enhancement* 32, 20–21.

DeFronzo, R. A. and Ferrannini, E. (1991). "Insulin Resistance: A multifaceted syndrome responsible for NIDDM, obesity, hypertension, dyslipidemia, and atherosclerotic cardiovascular disease." *Diabetes Care* 14 (3), 173–94.

Denker, P. S. and Pollock, V. E. (1992). "Fasting serum insulin levels in essential hypertension." *Archives of Internal Medicine* 152, 1649–51.

Eliahou, H. E. et al. (1981). "Body weight reduction necessary to attain normotension in the overweight hypertensive patient." *International Journal of Obesity* 5 (Suppl. 1), 157–63.

Endre, T. et al. (1994). "Insulin resistance is coupled to low fitness in normotensive men with a family history of hypertension." *Journal of Hypertension* 12, 81–88.

Ferrannini, E. et al. (1987). "Insulin resistance in essential hypertension." *New England Journal of Medicine* 317 (6), 350–57.

Fidelman, M. L. et al. (1982). "Intracellular pH mediates action of insulin of glycolysis in frog skeletal muscle." *American Journal of Physiology* 242, C87–93.

Flack, J. M. and Sowers, J. R. (1991). "Epidemiological and clinical aspects of insulin resistance and hyperinsulinemia." *American Journal of Medicine* 91 (Suppl. 1A), I1S–21S.

Welborn, T. A. and Frazer (1966). "Serum-insulin in essential hypertension and in peripheral vascular disease." *Lancet* 1, 1336–37.

Grady, D. (February 23, 1997). "Diet-diabetes link reported." *New York Times,* B12.

Haffner, S. M. et al. (1992). "Prospective analysis of the insulin-resistance syndrome (syndrome X)." *Diabetes* 41 (6), 715–22.

Jenkins, D. J. et al. (1981). "Glycemic index of foods: a physiologic basis for carbohydrate exchange." *American Journal of Clinical Nutrition* 34, 362–66.

Jenkins, D. J. et al. (1983). "The glycemic index of foods tested in diabetic patients: A new basis for carbohydrate exchange favoring the use of legumes." *Diabetologia* 24, 257–64.

Kannel, W. B. (1995). "Framingham study insights into hypertensive risk of cardiovascular disease." *Hypertension Research* 18, 181–96.

Kaplan, N. M. (1989). "The deadly quartet: Upper-body obesity, glucose intolerance, hypertriglyceridemia, and hypertension." *Archives of Internal Medicine* 149, 1512–20.

Karam, J. H. (1992). "Type II diabetes and syndrome X. Pathogenesis and glycemic management." *Endocrinology and Metabolism Clinics of North America* 21 (2), 329–50.

Knowler, W. C. et al. (1995). "Preventing non-insulin-dependent diabetes." *Diabetes* 44, 483–88.

Laitinen, J. (1994). "Metabolic and dietary determinants of serum lipids in obese patients with recently diagnosed non-insulin-dependent diabetes." *Annals of Medicine* 26, 119–24.

Langes, K. et al. (1995). "The significance of insulin resistance and hyperlipidemia in microvascular angina (syndrome X)." *Zeitschrift Fur Kardiologie* 84 (3), 180–89.

Lichtenstein, M. J. et al. (1987). "Sex hormones, insulin, lipids, and prevalent ischemic heart disease." *American Journal of Epidemiology* 126, 647–57.

Lindahl, B. et al. (1993). "High serum insulin, insulin resistance, and their associations with cardiovascular risk factors: The northern Sweden MONICA population study." *Journal of Internal Medicine* 234, 263–70.

Modan, M. et al. (1984). "Insulin resistance: A condition linking hypertension, glucose intolerance, obesity and Na+ K+ imbalance [Abstract]." *Israeli Medical Science* 20, 292.

———. (1985). "Hyperinsulinemia: A link between hypertension, obesity and glucose intolerance." *Journal of Clinical Investigating* 75, 809–17.

Moore, R. D. (1985). "The case for intracellular pH in insulin action." In M. P. Czech (Ed.), *Molecular Basis of Insulin Action.* New York: Plenum, 145–70.

Moore, R. D., Fidelman, M. L., Seeholzer, S. H. (1979). "Correlation between insulin action upon glycolysis and change in intracellular pH." *Biochemical and Biophysical Research Communications* Ret Cm 91, 905–10.

National Institute of Diabetes and Digestive and Kidney Diseases (1996). *Diabetes in America,* 2d ed. Bethesda, MD: NIDDK.

Pell, S. and D'Alonzo, C. A. (1967). "Some aspects of hypertension in diabetes mellitus." *Journal of the American Medical Association* 202, 104–10.

Pollare, T. H. et al. (1990). "Insulin resistance is a characteristic feature of primary hypertension independent of obesity." *Metabolism* 39 (2), 167–74.

Puska, P. et al. (1983). "Controlled, randomized trial of the effect of dietary fat on blood pressure." *Lancet* 1, 5–9.

Reaven, G. M. (1988). "Role of insulin resistance in human disease." *Diabetes* 37, 1595–1607.

———. (1991). "Insulin resistance, hyperinsulinemia, and hypertriglyceridemia in the etiology and clinical course of hypertension." *American Journal of Medicine* 90 (Suppl. 2A), 7S–12S.

———. (1994). "Syndrome X." *Clinical Diabetes* 3–4, 32–25.

Reaven, G. M. et al. (1967). "Role of insulin in endogenous hypertriglyceridemia." *Journal of Clinical Investigation* 46, 1756–67.

Reiser, S. et al. (1981). "Serum insulin and glucose in hyperinsulinemic subjects fed three different levels of sucrose." *American Journal of Clinical Nutrition* 34, 2348–58.

Salmeron, J. et al. (1997). "Dietary fiber, glycemic load, and risk of non-insulin-dependent diabetes mellitus in women." *Journal of the American Medical Association* 277, 472–77.

Singer, P. et al. (1985). "Postprandial hyperinsulinemia in patients with mild essential hypertension." *Hypertension* 7, 182–86.

Uusitupa, M. J. (1994). "Fructose in the diabetic diet." *American Journal of Clinical Nutrition* 59, 753S–57S.

Vaverkova, H. et al. (1993). "Reaven's metabolic syndrome X in the families of individuals with premature cerebrovascular attacks." *Vnitrni Lekarstvi* 39 (8), 745–54.

Weber, M. A. et al. (1991). "Cardiovascular and metabolic characteristics of hypertension." *American Journal of Medicine* 91 (Suppl. 1A), 4S–10S.

Weidmann, P. (1995). "Insulin resistance in hypertension." *Journal of Hypertension* (Suppl. 13), S65–S72.

Weidmann, P. et al. (1995). "Insulin resistenz und arterielle Hypertonie." *Herz* 20 (1), 16–32.

Welborn, T. A. et al. (1966). "Serum-insulin in essential hypertension and in peripheral vascular disease." *Lancet* 1, 1336–37.

Wirth, A. (1995). "Nichtmedikamentose therapie des metabolishen syndroms." *Herz* 20 (1), 56–59.

Wolever, T. M. et al. (1991). "The glycemic index: Methodology and clinical implications." *American Journal of Clinical Nutrition* 54, 846–54.

———. (1993). "Glycemic index of fruits and fruit products in patients with diabetes." *International Journal of Food Sciences and Nutrition* 43, 205–12.

Wolever, T. M. and Jenkins, D. J. (1986). "The use of the glycemic index in predicting the blood glucose response to mixed meals." *American Journal of Clinical Nutrition* 43, 167–72.

Wright, J. V. (1990). "The glucose-insulin tolerance test and its relevance to essential hypertension and HDL/LDL cholesterol abnormalities." *International Clinical Nutrition Review* 10, 381–83.

WATER

Batmanghelidj, F. (1987). "Pain: A need for paradigm change." *Anti-cancer Research* 7, 971–90.

————. (1995). *Your Body's Many Cries for Water.* Falls Church, VA: Global Health Solutions.

Craun, G. (1988). "Surface water supplies and health." *JAWWA* 40.

Espiner, E. A. (1987). "The effect of stress on salt and water balance." *Bailliere's Clinical Endocrinology and Metabolism* 1 (2).

Goldstein, D. J. et al. (1978). "Increase in mast cell number and altered vascular permeability in thirsty rats." *Life Sciences* 60, 1591–1602.

Herwart, B. L. et al. (1992). "Outbreaks of waterborne disease in the US: 1989–90." *JAWWA* 29.

Humes, H. D. (1986). "Disorders of water metabolism, fluids and electrolytes." In Kokko and Tannen and Saunders (Eds.), 118–49.

Morris, K. (1997). "Water, water, everywhere—but is it safe to drink?" *Lancet* 350, 567.

Morris, R. D. et al. (1992). "Chlorination, chlorination by-products, and cancer: A meta-analysis." *American Journal of Public Health* 82 (7), 955–63.

Robertson, R. P. and Chin, M. (1973). "A role for prostaglandin E in defective insulin secretion and carbohydrate intolerance in diabetes mellitus." *Journal of Clinical Investigations* 60, 747–53.

Index